Instructor's Guide to

Critical Thinking: Cases in Respiratory Care

Kathleen J. Wood, MED, RRT
Assistant Professor of Respiratory Care
Massasoit Community College
Brockton, Massachusetts

With contributions by Lawrence A. Dahl, EdD, RRT
Program Coordinator, Respiratory Therapy Technology
Hawkeye Institute of Technology, Waterloo, Iowa

F. A. Davis Company
1915 Arch Street
Philadelphia, PA 19103
http://www.fadavis.com

Last digit indicates print number: 10 9 8 7 6 5 4 3 2 1

Instructors in educational institutions who have adopted *Critical Thinking: Cases in Respiratory Care* for use as a textbook may freely reproduce material from this instructor's guide for educational purposes only.

Printed in the United States of America

ISBN 0-8036-0265-0

Contents

EXPERT OPINIONS FOR CHAPTER 2

1. There are six core skills in CT: interpretation, analysis, evaluation, inference, explanation, and self-regulation. Each of these terms can be modified in many ways, such as when "inference" refers to drawing conclusions as opposed to querying evidence. Although each term is precise to its own definition, there is plenty of room to elaborate on the "bigger" definitions. There is also a group of terms, called dispositions, that modify the critical thinker. These dispositions, referring to a person's character, include truthseeking, open-mindedness, analytical, systematic, inquisitive, self-confident, and mature. Not all critical thinkers will reflect all of these qualities at all times. These dispositions represent the overall picture of the ideal critical thinker.

2. This is a self-evaluation exercise. One may view his or her own use of each CT skill and evaluate the level of performance on each. CT may be enhanced by practice, particularly within a specific discipline, like RC. Such practice strategies include working within a problem-based learning environment, performing research, participating in debates, engaging in structured controversy, analyzing literature, or any combination of the items listed in Table 2-3. It should not be excluded that the individual may find his or her own route to enhancing CT as well.

3. This is a self-evaluation exercise. You could invent a scenario where you were required to make a judgment, such as in developing a weaning schedule for a mechanically ventilated patient. Then you could evaluate how CT would guide the decisions.

4. Refer to your situation and make inference. You are free to create and bound to learn.

5. You should examine your example and cite specific instances of CT. To provide some example, I will examine a generic situation:

   CT is in constant use within the profession of RC, where problems of several natures await the start of each day. RCPs are called to use all of the skills and subskills continuously. The outstanding practitioners exemplify the dispositions associated with CT, for they are a model of excellence. I am never more proud of being an RCP than when I see a fellow professional carefully analyze a problem, query evidence, assess the situation fully, clarify the problem, and then be so kind as to explain the whole thing to a coworker. As this kind of situation occurs each critically thinking RCP will continuously assess his or her own performance and adjust as needed.

6. This is personal choice... obviously the author has a certain affinity for the problem-based learning route! You should elaborate on your choice. This process breeds CT growth.

7. Same as above.

8. To understand the process of controversy, as displayed in Figure 2-3, one needs to proceed in a systematic fashion. This logical process proceeds from making inferences and interpreting data, to feeling confused when conflict begins, to reasoning things out, to using resources, and finally to reorganizing one's thoughts while viewing the whole process. The end result of such thought organization is sound judgment formation, based on reasoning and evidence.

9 and 10. These are personal choice and self-evaluative exercises.

11. Novice RCPs tend to be very inquisitive and very connected to the rules and guidelines of the practice. Experts will also abide by these same guides, while at the same time depending on their own experi-

ences. This body of experience is what enables the expert to have greater insight and capacity for predicting outcomes to a reasonable degree.

12. Experts and novices share interest in their common subject and relate to one another in a complimentary way. For instance, when a novice begins his or her first professional job, it is often the resident expert that enjoys the excitement and satisfaction of performing the duties of preceptor, or guide.

References

1. Scanlan, C: Fundamentals of Respiratory Care, ed 6. Mosby, St. Louis, 1995.
2. Kacmarak, R: Foundations of Respiratory Care. Churchill Livingstone, 1992.

EXPERT OPINIONS FOR CHAPTER 3

1. Systematicity promotes effective assessment skill proficiency by assuring consistency and by reducing the risk of overlooking significant findings.

2. In general, arguments should present evidence and reasons for one's own preference (e.g., check lists, head to toe)

3. CT assures quality in assessment by assuring that meaningful relationships are drawn between assessments and patient status (or problem status). As outcomes of CT, information gathering and decision making combine to facilitate the RC process in general.

4. The advantages of using reference materials during the clinical practice of RC include the availability of information, updates, guidelines, new findings, definitions, values, and other such cornerstone necessities. The disadvantages would include the use of time required to use the materials (reading, going to a computer station, etc.). However, the availability of information nearly always outweighs the cost in time of accessing it. Still, in times of emergency, direct care would take clear precedence over the desire to check sources.

5. When information is taken in, it then becomes a factor in the thinking process. When unexpected findings are uncovered, they become clues for further assessment. For instance, if during routine chest examination moist rales are heard diffusely and the patient is experiencing some shortness of breath, a chest radiograph to rule in/out congestive heart failure may be indicated.

6. Unusual findings create a focus for the planning process. They present clues to problems or conditions that may in themselves require specialized care.

7. There is a wide range of answers to this one. They should make for interesting responses.

8. Such tools as checklists and flowsheets minimize the costs and risks of patient care and maximize the process. Incorporation of all CT skills serves as a comprehensive enhancement to care as well. (For instance, systematic assessment cuts down on oversight.)

9. Knowledge of standards within a special population affects the delivery and quality of care rendered. Standards that are different and thus may require adjustment include height/weight norms, laboratory values, vital sign ranges, and physical examination norms (like grunting in the neonate).

10. Some cultural beliefs related to medicine include:
    - Use of food as a healing tool
    - Herbal therapies
    - Prayer or ritual use
    - The power of positive thinking
    - The use of healing touch

    Some ways to enhance your own cultural expansion include reading, researching, meeting people of other cultures, and observation.

11. The outcome of any case depends on the assessments that are made during the case. The assessments serve as the measure of success or failure in care.

12. High-level assessment skill promote better outcomes by assuring consistency, completeness, and accuracy in information gathering and decision making.

EXPERT OPINIONS FOR CHAPTER 4

1. Evaluation is a subskill of critical thinking. The other subskills are integrated with evaluation.

2. Example (but creativity is desirable):

    Name:
    Diagnosis:
    Physician:
    Is oxygen therapy indicated?
    Is oxygen in use?
    Is oxygen set up properly?
    Is prescription appropriately followed?

3. To assess the validity of such an instrument, one would need to determine if the tool did, in fact, do what it was supposed to do. Checking with other such instruments for format and requesting other professionals for critique would ensure this. To assess reliability, one would need to observe the findings produced by the tool and see that they were repeatable over time.

4. An evaluation system generates excellence in service by broadening the overall perspective. By allowing users and deliverers of a service to have input, interventions can be created and thus quality improved.

5. This may serve as a good research opportunity, where students may seek the input of local RC managers or personnel departments. An overall tool would include:

    * Evaluation criteria (self-evaluation)
    * Peer evaluation (supervisor evaluation)
    * Competency checks (specific skills)
    * Client survey attached to the above information

6. The merit of using such an integrated evaluation system includes the potential for individual and departmental improvement as well as team building. The negative points of such a system would include the resource requirement of tracking and maintaining such a system.

7. A logical argument should be based on evidence such as is found in question 6 (improvement, team building, etc.).

8. Departmental inservices may be designed according to areas of general staff need.

9. Individual responses will vary but should include the example, an evaluation, and the use of evidence in judgments.

10. Refer to question 9.

11. Negative occurrences may be used to improve departmental quality by allowing prevention strategies to be discussed and implemented.

12 and 13. Such input may allow for improvement and tailoring in service to clients' needs and wants.

14. Process evaluations monitor ongoing activities. Impact evaluations monitor the effectiveness of the service in producing a favorable response. Outcome evaluations measure the degree to which stated objectives are met.

15. Answers should include focus on audits or checklists, assessments of need, indicators of problems, and criteria featuring critical incidents. Timelines should be realistic in that they neither require excessive time expenditure nor produce unreasonable deadlines.

16. All staff should be involved in quality maintenance in an RC department.

17. Answers will vary, but evaluate based on the inclusion of criteria in making projections.

18. Feedback generated through the evaluation process directs the outcome of any plan.

19. Answers should include notation of the fact that RCPs are highly responsible in outcome management of their patients.

EXPERT OPINIONS FOR CHAPTER 5

1 and 2.

Guideline Topic	Indication	Assessments of Outcome

Ventilator checks	- prior to obtaining ABG
	- following parameter changes
	- following an acute change in change
	- prior to obtaining hemodynamic
	   or bedside pulmonary function data
	- anytime that ventilator performance is
	   questionable
		- preventions of untoward incidents
		- warning of impending events
		- assure that proper ventilator settings
		   are maintained according to
		   physician's order

Oxygen therapy	- documented hypoxemia (PaO2 <60; SaO2<90% in adults) - suspected hypoxemia - severe trauma - acute myocardial infarction - short-term therapy (postanesthesia)	- adequate response to therapy

Incentive spirometry	- presence of conditions predisposing to
	   the development of pulmonary
	   atelectasis
	- presence of atelectasis
	- presence of a restrictive lung defect
	   associated with quadraplegia
	   and/or dysfunctional diaphragm
		- absence of or improvement in signs of
		   atelectasis
		- improved inspiratory muscle perfor-
		   mance

3. A decision tree is a graphic illustration of a decision-making process that is specific to an event. Such tools are usually incorporated into protocol plans in order to assist in making treatment choices. They help to maintain consistency in the RC planning process, as well as offer cues to options of care.

4. Incentive spirometry decision tree:

Incentive Spirometry

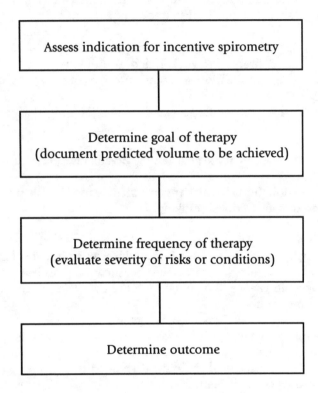

5. This question requires individual research.

EXPERT OPINIONS FOR CHAPTER 6

1. Time management is an essential skill for RCPs to hone. It fosters efficiency and safety in the clinical setting. Poor time-management skill may lead to poor job performance.

2. Answers should allude to the following general problems associated with lack of good time management in an organization. Poor delivery of services, lack of coordination of services and goods, and general chaos of the structure of an organization are some outcomes of poor time structure.

3. Time structure is correlated with sense of purpose, self-esteem, standing, optimism, and efficient study habits.

4. The essential skills of time management are goal setting, organizing, and regulating the process.

5. This is a self-evaluative question, but potential answers include use of tools such as lists, schedules, computer aids, notes, and of course critical thinking.

6. Prioritizing of care involves careful assessment of need. Those in greatest need (i.e., those at the greatest risk) are given immediate needed care. Therefore all life-saving care must be administered as a top priority. When one patient is stabilized, the next may be cared for. This is a basic triage strategy. Quality care is assured by maintenance of high level standard practice, which is performed on a continuous basis and evaluated intermittently.

7. Effectiveness may be measured in terms of initial goals. In a case such as this where the time for initiating aerosolized medication treatments should be reduced, effectiveness could be measured in view of the stated goal. An example of such a goal could be: Response time between request for emergency department nebulizer treatments and initiation of the treatment will be reduced by 15% within 1 month's time. Suggestions as to how time could be reduced should be discussed and action plans implemented. As an outcome evaluation the situation should be assessed by the month's end and an evaluation made. (Were changes effective in achieving the goal or not?) Efficiency may be measured simply by measuring the previous average time of response to the present response time and stating the difference.

8. Time conflict results when time demands from one part of your life, interfere with time demands in another area (e.g., you must stay late at work when you already have a dinner engagement). This type of conflict may result in dissatisfaction, frustration, or even depression.

9. Prevention of time conflict may occur via use of goal setting, prioritizing, limit setting, negotiating, and communicating.

10. This is a self-evaluation question.

11. In a patient/client care setting, immediate needs must always be addressed, even at the risk of putting off a long-term project.

12. Potential outcomes of time management include minimizing stress, higher self-esteem, lower depression rates, production of a more positive outlook on the future, improved efficiency, improved job satisfaction, and increased effectiveness. An argument in favor of using time management skills related to producing these outcomes should be made.

13. Both the efficiency and effectiveness of an organization are related to time management. On an individual level, multiple enhancements to one's life are apparent. (See question 12 for specifics.)

References

1. Bond, JF and Feather, NT: Some correlates of structure and purpose in the use of time. Journal of Personality and Social Psychology 55:327, 1988.
2. Resohazy, R: Recent social developments and changes in attitudes to time. ISSJ 107, 1986.
3. O'Driscoll, M et al: Time devoted to job and off-job activities, interrole conflict, and affective experiences. Journal of Applied Psychology 77:277, 1992.

EXPERT OPINIONS FOR CHAPTER 7

1. Yes.

2. Risk factors include dyspnea and history of smoking 2pks/day × 18 yr. Dyspnea may contribute to respiratory distress during treatment. It may also obscure the respiratory practitioner's ability to identify new problems associated with treatment. Smoking is related to poorer postoperative recovery and is clearly related to lung cancers.

3. These risks may predispose the patient to pulmonary and/or cardiovascular complications, postoperatively.

4. Postoperative atelectasis or pneumonia are quite possible. Bronchospasm is also possible.

5. The patient should receive preoperative teaching in incentive spirometry, deep breathing, and coughing. Chest physical therapy procedures may also be discussed. Thorough explanation and evaluation should occur to foster compliance with postoperative routines.

6. No.

7. Pulmonary hemorrhage, atelectasis, pneumonia, or cardiovascular compromise may occur.

8. A pulmonary hygiene regimen including incentive spirometry, coughing, chest percussion, and vibration could be initiated.

9. Bronchial adenoma is a benign neoplasm having a glandular structure and is thought to arise from the mucus glands of the bronchi. Although termed "adenoma," this tumor is recognized as being low-grade malignancy. It occurs equally in both sexes and has a prolonged course. The endobronchial portion of the tumor dilates and obstructs the bronchus. Metastasis is infrequent.

   Associated respiratory clinical findings include cough, dyspnea, hemoptysis, chest pain, wheezing, and sputum production. Difficulty swallowing, weight loss, malaise, and joint or bone pain are included among nonrespiratory findings.

   Physical findings at diagnosis and complications associated with the disease are frequently related to bronchial obstruction and include localized wheezing, atelectasis, pneumonia, and pleural effusion.

10.

Interventions	Assessments
Incentive spirometry q1 hr.	Chest radiograph.
Oxygen via nebulizer postoperatively.	Discontinue when ABGs are within normal limits and patient demonstrates spontaneous coughing ability.
Physical observation.	Reassess and evaluate plan q 24 hr unless patient condition indicates change in plan.

11. Positive responses include maintenance of oxygenation and ventilation as assessed using ABG data, clear breath sounds, and clear chest radiograph. Also the presence of a strong and clear cough would indicate a positive response.

12. Responses that indicate lack of success would include poor chest radiograph, crackles and wheezing, congested coughing, and poor ABG results.

13. It is complete for now.

14. Not at this time.

15. IPPB is indicated by day 3, because of the lack of successful outcome in using incentive spirometry. On day 2 atelectasis is observed. The patient's inspiratory capacity is also significantly lower than predicted and blood gases reveal compromised oxygenation (with PaO_2 of 80 while on 50% oxygen). Also temperature is present, as may occur with atelectasis or with infection.

16. This modification to the therapeutic plan is indicated.

17. Example order: IPPB to be administered q 3 hr to achieve tidal volumes >550 mL. during treatment.

18. Objective: promote resolution of atelectasis.

19. Outcome would be assessed by chest radiograph and auscultation, while still monitoring vital signs, oxygenation, and general physical observations.

20. Oxygen therapy is regulated appropriately. Oximetry and partial pressure of arterial oxygen were the chief assessments used to guide the therapy.

EXPERT OPINIONS FOR CHAPTER 8

1. The patient is having an acute exacerbation of asthma with poor ventilatory exchange.

2. The assessments that will be used to guide the RC plan include heart rate, respiratory rate, peak expiratory flow rate (PEFR), breath sounds, observation of accessory muscle use, blood pressure, level of dyspnea, level of consciousness, color, oxygen saturation, and subjective statements.

3. The plan is appropriate. Steroid therapy may be initiated at this time if desired.

4. Findings in this case according to severity at this point:

    PEFR: Moderately severe

    Vital signs: RR, HR, and BP are elevated and warrant close monitoring. These findings correlate with hypoxemia. Pulsus paradoxus >12 mmHg indicates moderate/severe airflow obstruction.

    Physical appearance: Marked use of accessory muscles indicates significant ventilatory impairment. Distant breath sounds are an ominous sign, indicating poor aeration. I & E wheezing represent bronchoconstriction. Facial flushing, diaphoresis and trembling may represent perfusion problems and anxiety, although trembling may be associated with albuterol use. Dark circles under the eyes represent fatigue and fluid depletion.

5. Therapeutic indications for:

    Oxygen therapy: SpO2 of 90%, elevated HR and BP, accompanied by the signs of bronchoconstriction noted, indicate the need for oxygen.

    Nebulized albuterol: Auscultation findings, PEFR, oxygenation status, and physical appearance indicate the need for this bronchodilator intervention.

6. Therapeutic objectives:

    Oxygen therapy: to improve oxygen indices, with PaO2 > 85mmHg and/or SpO2 > 95%.

    Albuterol nebulizer: to improve airflow obstruction as indicated by improved breath sounds, limited use of accessory muscles, no dyspnea, improved color and O2 saturation, as well as improved PEFR to > 70% predicted.

7. Changes in arterial blood gases and pulse oximetry as well as vital signs and physical observation will be used to evaluate the effects of oxygen therapy. Changes in PEFR, accessory muscle use, auscultation, physical appearance, and vital signs will be used to evaluate the albuterol treatment.

8. Subcutaneous epinephrine may be given if the patient is unlikely to benefit from aerosol (e.g., decreased consciousness, intolerance of aerosol, intolerance of the nebulizer, etc.) One must bear in mind, however, the likely effects this medication will have on heart rate and blood pressure.

    Intravenous or aerosolized corticosteroids may be given their antt-inflammatory effect. These drugs also enhance or potentiate the effect of (-adrenergic drugs such as albuterol.

    Intravenous aminophylline is advocated by some as a drug of first choice, followed by adrenergics as indicated. Others feel that nebulizing adrenergics is more desirable, as they are more rapid and the process is less invasive.

Nebulized anticholinergic drugs (atropine, ipratropium bromide), frequently in conjunction with adrenergic drugs, may be given for their additive effects. Ipratropium bromide in particular has minimal cardiovascular effects and may be given in place of adrenergics to sensitive patients. The bronchodilating effects of anticholinergics is somewhat less than that of adrenergics, however.

9. All of the following are signs of improvement: Breath sounds are more audible.   Subjective statement is positive. SpO2 increases to 95% and PEFR improves to 65% of baseline. Pulsus paradoxus lessens, respiratory frequency decreases to 32, and no adverse effects are noted.

10. According to the Guidelines for the Diagnosis and Management of Asthma, the choice to continue reatment, as well as consider admission is an optimal choice, given that PEFR is still <70% of baseline.

11. The current ABG, drawn at 9:20AM with an FiO2 of .21, reveals mild respiratory alkalosis (hyperventilation) and moderate hypoxemia and indicates that a significant correlation exists between arterial oxygen saturation and oximetry values.

12. At this point in the case the PEFR has improved to 70% of baseline, indicating a positive outcome so far. The patient's HR and RR have decreased and subjective statements indicate progression of status.

13. The third treatment was indicated according to current guidelines. The primary indication was the PEFR < 70%.

14. The treatment preceded the increase in PEFR to >75% of predicted baseline and therefore is likely to have caused the positive outcome.

15. At this time the patient is sufficiently improved to warrant discharge. Patient education, medication, and follow-up are essential to optimal care.

16. Criteria supporting discharge at this time are:

    PEFR>79% predicted
    Stable vital signs, within age norms.
    SpO2>95%
    Observation of physical appearance indicates patient stability without dyspnea.

17. Discharge plan:

    Indication for therapy: Acute exacerbation of asthma

    Therapeutic objectives: 1. The patient will demonstrate clear breath sounds and maintain her
                                       PEFR > 75% of baseline value.
                                   2. The patient will demonstrate a clear understanding of prevention
                                       and treatment of asthma symptoms.

    Interventions: 1. Inhaled albuterol.
                                   2. Patient education.

    Outcome evaluations: 1. Auscultation, daily PEFR monitoring, and symptom recording
                                   2. Written and verbal assessment of understanding key learning
                                       content

18. Educational objectives:

    1. The patient will demonstrate clear understanding of:
        - Asthma's definition and goals of therapy
        - The signs and symptoms of asthma
        - Characteristic changes in the airways of asthma patients and the role of medication

- Asthma triggers and avoidance
- Treatment
- Emotional elements in asthma control
- Use of written guidelines
- Use of written diaries
- Correct use of inhalers, therapies, and peak flow meter
- Criteria for premedicating to prevent onset of symptoms
- Optimal use of home peak flow rate monitoring
- Evaluation of therapeutic results
- Family understanding and support

2. Communication with the child's school will occur and continue.

3. The patient will demonstrate self-management skills by maintaining documentation of progress, adhering to the RC plan, and demonstrating proper technical skills (i.e., PEFR monitoring, MDI use).

19. The educational objectives should be evaluated by immediate caregiver assessment incorporating demonstration, question and answer, and discussion. Follow-up should consist of the same with home surveys, visits, and telephone checks.

20. Common triggers in asthma:

    Allergens and irritants
    Upper respiratory infections, usually viral
    Bacterial otitis and sinusitis
    Influenza and pneumococcal pulmonary infections
    Exercise
    Cold environment
    Seasonal changes

21. In treating extrinsic asthma, the identification of provoking and exacerbating factors is extremely important. Avoidance of these factors or immunotherapy may dramatically reduce the need for additional therapy.

    In cases that involve bacterial infection, rapid and thorough antibiotic therapy may prevent an extended course of therapy.

    Underlying emotional problems may be at least partly responsible for asthmatic attacks in some individuals. Appropriate psychiatric counseling may be of benefit to these patients.

    Because each patient may be thought of as being unique, education of the patient about the disease and individual exacerbating and complicating factors is important. Recruitment of the patient as an active participant in therapy may offer the best hope of decreasing the incidence of severe episodes.

Reference

1. National Asthma Education Program Expert Panel Report Executive Summary: Guidelines for the Diagnosis and Management of Asthma. National Heart, Lung and Blood Institute, National Institutes of Health. US Department of Health and Human Services. June 1991, NIH Publication No. 91-3042A.

EXPERT OPINIONS FOR CHAPTER 9

1. Assessments noted in this case that are typically associated with the diagnosis of AIDS are malaise, cachexia, lymphadenopathy, history of infection, and history of the diagnosis. Dyspnea, orthopnea, cough, and dull percussion notes are significant for pulmonary infection in AIDS.

2. | Intervention | Indication |
    |---|---|
    | O_2 therapy | SpO_2= 90% |
    | Hypertonic saline via USN | Need for sputum induction |

3. The RLL consolidation is suspicious for pneumonia. The miliary nodular pattern may be representative of several different types of infection, thus radiography alone will not serve as a differential diagnostic.[1]

4. Expected outcomes for interventions:

Intervention	Outcome	Evaluation Tools
O_2 therapy	Normoxia	ABG, oximetry, ECG, and appearance/color
Hypertonic saline via USN	Sputum induction	Observation of sputum production and retrieval of sample; auscultation

5. The mode of oxygen delivery is determined by the patient demonstrating hypoxemia. The cannula is chosen for its low-flow capability, as higher flows and FiO2's are not desirable at this point in the case.

6. Essential laboratory data include:

Test	Rationale
ABG	Assessment of oxygenation and ventilation
CBC	Assesses erythrocyte count (RBC), leukocytes (WBC), and platelet (thrombocyte) count. Also assesses differential counts—most notably lymphocyte counts.
Tuberculin skin test	Assesses presence of tuberculosis infection (although many HIV-infected patients who have TB infection do not have positive PPD tests).[2]
Sputum analysis	Culture and sensitivity may determine the infecting organism and its likely sensitivity

7. Precautions necessary for optimal patient care as well as protection of both the patient and health-care worker are summatively demonstrated in the practice of universal precautions.

8. The RC plan:

Indications	Objectives	Interventions	Expected Outcomes
1. Hypoxemia	Increase SpO_2 > 90% Increase PaO_2 > 60	O_2 therapy	SpO_2 > 90%

2. Need for sputum sample while patient has nonproductive cough.	Obtain sputum sample.	Hypertonic saline via USN.	Specimen obtained with no adverse effect to patient and by the least invasive means appropriate

9. Bronchoscopy is indicated by the failure of USN treatment to assist the patient in sputum production and ultimately retrieval of a sample.[3]

10. Objective for bronchoscopy in this case—obtain bronchoalveolar sputum sample for evaluation.

11. The primary role of the bronchoscopic assistant includes preparation and monitoring of the patient, assisting with the procedure, handling specimens, post-procedure care of the patient, maintenance of the bronchoscopy equipment, and record keeping.[3]

12. Checklist for assembling and checking bronchoscopic equipment: [3,4]

Supplies and Equipment

Fiberoptic bronchoscope, cleaned and of appropriate size for patient.
Bronchoscopic light source, working.
Video/photographic equipment if needed.
Cytology brushes, forceps, transbronchial aspiration needles, retrieval baskets—all compatible with scope size.
Specimen collection devices and fixatives.
Specimen containers
Syringes
Sterile needles
Isotonic saline
Bite block
Laryngoscope
Endotracheal tubes of various sizes
Thoracostomy set/tray
Venous access equipment

Monitors

Oximeter
ECG apparatus
Sphygmomanometer
Radiation badges for personnel
Stethoscope
Oxygen equipment
Swivel adaptors
Resuscitation equipment
Vacuum system and suction equipment
Infection control devices
Fluoroscopy equipment
Laser equipment if applicable
Protease enzymatic agent for cleaning before disinfection process
Disinfection or sterilizing agent
Adequate ventilation in environment

Medications

Lidocaine 1%, 2%, 4%
Sedative agent 30–40 min prior to procedure

IV sedative immediately prior to procedure
Benzodiazepine antagonist, narcotic antagonist
Sterile nonbacteriostatic isotonic saline
Vasoconstrictor for bleeding (epinephrine)
Inhaled beta agonist (albuterol, metaproterenol)
Water-soluble lubricant
Emergency and resuscitation drugs as needed

Procedures

Perform leak test on scope
Check bronchoscope channel integrity
Assure proper cleaning procedures
Assure smooth operation of retrieval devices
Perform patient monitoring:
    Level of consciousness
    Medications delivered, dosage, route, and time
    Subjective response
    Vital signs
    SpO_2 & FiO_2
    Ventilatory parameters if appropriate to situation
    Lavage volumes
    Document site of biopsies, washings, and tests on samples
    Periodic postprocedure check of patient condition for 24–48 hours after procedure (fever, chest
        pain, discomfort, dyspnea, wheezing, hemoptysis, or new findings—ADVISE outpatients of same)

Maintain Records

Quality assessment indicators
Document monitors and findings
Identify equipment used
Annual assessment of institutional or department bronchoscopy procedure
Maintain infection control standards and procedures

13. Adverse effects associated with bronchoscopy are adverse medication effects, hypoxemia, hypercarbia, wheezing, hypotension, laryngospasm, bradycardia (or other vagal reactions), trauma including epistaxis, pneumothorax, and hemoptysis, increased airway resistance, death, infection risk for patient, health care workers and others in local environment, and cross-contamination of the specimens or equipment.[3]

14. Contingency plans for negative events may include:

    - use of proper antagonist or appropriate support and treatment for medication effects
    - assure oxygenation and ventilation to support patient to prevent/treat hypoxemia and hypercarbia
    - institute bronchodilator therapy for wheezing
    - provide appropriate regulatory therapy for hypotension (medication, fluids, position)
    - maintain airway patency via pharmacological or mechanical routes
    - treat bradycardia as needed (i.e.: atropine)
    - facilitate bleeding control via medication, cold irrigation or direct pressure
    - provide patent airway to maintain lower airway resistance
    - be vigilantly prepared to institute both basic and advanced life support measures
    - adhere to infection control standards & policies
    - maintain strict adherence to cleaning and disinfection policies

15. Mr. Chan's emotional state represents both positive and negative conditions. On the positive side Mr. Chan is communicating his feelings and this must never be overlooked in significance. On the negative

side he is feeling poorly about his condition and expresses fear. While each health care provider will have differing responses in such a case, an overall strategy for dealing with grief and the dying process necessitates careful attention to one's existing attitudes toward death, current literature on the subject, and appropriate avenues for communicating with people in nonjudgmental and caring ways.[5]

16. Bronchospasm occurred in response to the procedure, thus necessitating a bronchodilator intervention. Other physiologic assessments indicate mild and probably transient changes associated with the procedure.

17. The CD-4 lymphocyte count of 155/mm^3 indicates the need for prophylactic therapy against pneumocystis carinii infection or reinfection. Such prophylaxis currently includes the combination or singular use of trimethoprim and sulfamethoxazole, dapsone, clindamycin, primaquine, atovaquone, trimetrexate, intravenous pentamidine, and aerosolized pentamidine. It is also likely in viewing the patient symptoms and this laboratory data that the current infection is caused by p.carinii, thus requiring the same medications as listed previously and possibly including the use of glucocorticosteroids to reduce pulmonary inflammation.[1]

18. At this point in the case the discontinuation of oxygen therapy should be considered, as no current indication exists. Continued monitoring and follow-up care are needed and Mr. Chan's emotional needs should be addressed in a health-care team format.

19. Monitoring plan:

> oximetry... spot checks for 24–48 hr.
> ECG postprocedure
> vital signs q 2–4 hr.
> subjective checks for pain/discomfort

20. Pulmonary problems and their associated radiographic patterns that are likely to be present in an AIDS patient include:

Pattern	Disease
Normal findings	*P. carinii* pneumonia
	Disseminated *Mycobacterium avium*-complex (MAC)
	Disseminated histoplasmosis
	Tuberculosis
	Kaposi's sarcoma
	Nonspecific interstitial pneumonitis
Diffuse reticulonodular infiltration	*P. carinii* pneumonia
	Disseminated tuberculosis
	Disseminated histoplasmosis
	Disseminated coccidioidomycosis
	Lymphocytic interstitial pneumonitis
	Nonspecific interstitial pneumonitis
	Kaposi's sarcoma
	Cryptococcosis
	Community-acquired bacterial pneumonia
	Strongyloidosis
	Respiratory syncytial virus pneumonia
	Atypical tuberculosis
	Lymphoma

Pattern	Disease
Focal airspace consolidation	*P. carinii* pneumonia
	Bacterial pneumonia
	Kaposi's sarcoma
	Cryptococcosis
	Legionellosis
	Mycoplasmal pneumonia
	Community-acquired bacterial pneumonitis
	Strongyloidosis
Primary upper lobe infiltrates	*P. carinii* pneumonia
	Tuberculosis
	Rhodococcus equi pneumonia
Adenopathy	*P. carinii* pneumonia
	Tuberculosis
	Disseminated MAC
	Kaposi's sarcoma
	Non-Hodgkin's lymphoma
	Cryptococcosis
Pleural effusion	Kaposi's sarcoma
	Tuberculosis
	Cryptococcosis
	Non-Hodgkin's lymphoma
Cavitations and pneumatoceles	Histoplasmosis
	P. carinii pneumonia
	Tuberculosis
	Rhodococcus equi pneumonia
	Strongyloidosis
Pneumothorax	*P. carinii* pneumonia

21. The CD-4 lymphocyte count of <200cells/mm^3 is a factor that predisposes an HIV positive individual to p.carinii infection. This level is also a predictor of the progression of HIV infection.[1]

22. Medications and actions:

   Trimethoprim-sulfamethoxazole: antimicrobial agent
   Prednisone: steroidal agent, antiinflammatory

23. The albuterol MDI treatment was indicated by the occurrence of post-bronchoscopy bronchoconstriction.

24. Team members and their roles:

   RCP:
       - coordinates/plans service and equipment with the durable medical equipment company
       - provides education and evaluation of treatment techniques, pathophysiology, breathing
         exercises, secretion clearance, and symptom recognition.

   Physician:
       - responsible for overseeing total care plan

   Nurse:
       - coordinates nursing services/plans

- provides education and evaluation of self-care strategies, medications, pathophysiology, and symptom recognition

Social worker:
- coordinates community services/plans
- provides education in accessing counseling
- assists in assessment of financial options

Note: any of the above members of the team may serve as team coordinator.

25. It is most likely that overlap exists between all of the roles described. It should also be clear that these roles are flexible in themselves. Professionals who are "cross-trained" in more than one area may accept more than one role in the health-care setting.

26. Key team members not listed include family members; the patient himself; a nutritionist; physical or occupational therapist; and community members such as friends, neighbors, and clergy.

27. Discharge plan:

Objectives:
- promote self-care
- provide support and enhance communication
- prevent opportunistic infection through education and behavioral modes
- control pulmonary symptoms

Expected outcomes:
- no readmission due to failure of plan
- long-term planning begins
- early recognition of symptoms facilitating early intervention
- wheezing is controlled

28. Guidelines for the nebulization of pentamidine prophylaxis are:
300 mg of pentamidine isethionate suspended in 6 mL of sterile water
Nebulized via the Respirgard II nebulizer (Marquest Medical Products, Englewood CO)[1]

Note: the current trend in prophylaxis for p. carinii is the use of Trimethoprim and sulfamethoxazole, while pentamidine aerosolization is generally used in the population of recipients who have sensitivity to sulfa.

29. As in any other educational pursuit, preparation for work with dying and grieving people requires careful study, practice, and consideration. There are considerable resources on the topics of death, grieving, and coping, some of which are listed in the reference section of this chapter. In an effort to oversimplify the scope of such a broad topic, it is always a sound strategy to enhance communication, whether learning about the dying process or participating in it.

References

1. Medin, D and Ognibene, F: Pulmonary disease in AIDS: Implications for respiratory care practitioners. Respiratory Care 40:832, 1995.
2. Hopewell, PC: Impact of human immunodeficiency virus infection on the epidemiology, clinical features, management and control of tuberculosis. Clin Infect Dis 15:540, 1992.
3. AARC clinical practice guidelines: Fiberoptic bronchoscopy assisting. Respiratory Care 38: 1173.
4. Brutinel, W and Cortese, D: Bronchoscopy. In Burton, G, Hodgkin, J, and Ward, J: Respiratory Care: A Guide to Clinical Practice, ed 3. JB Lippincott, Philadelphia, 1991, p 697.
5. Kubler-Ross, E: On Death and Dying. Macmillan Publishing, 1969.

EXPERT OPINIONS FOR CHAPTER 10

This case is easily integrated with laboratory or clinical practice in polysomnography and/or homecare, by assigning activities associated with the case. One such assignment might include participation in performing a sleep study and documenting lead placements, preparation steps, and scoring methods used. Another approach may place the learner in the homecare or hospital setting performing assessment on a patient with sleep apnea syndrome. Structured "in-class" dialogue strategies could focus on the incidence and prevalence of the problem and generate discussion concerning the need for intervention locally and nationally. This situation could generate many research questions such as: Is there a local need for a sleep lab? Do existing homecare companies provide the necessary services for this population and are the services distributed equally among companies or their "specialty" companies? and What is the average length (days, months, years) of service needed by OSAS patients in the community?

1. Assessments that identify sleep apnea syndrome in this initial report are daytime fatigue, agitation, AM headache, snoring, obesity, prominent p-waves, and peripheral edema.

2. There are three basic categories of sleep apnea: obstructive, which is caused by closure of the pharyngeal airway during inspiration[1]; central, which is caused by lack of central respiratory drive; and mixed, which is a combination of both.

3. Corpulmonale.

4. Polysomnography is the collective process of monitoring and recording physiologic data during sleep. Variables monitored include EEG (electroencephalogram—global neural activity), EOG (electrooculogram—eye movements), EMG (electromyogram—muscular activity/ movement), ECG (electrocardiograph—cardiac rhythm and rate), respiratory effort (numerous methods available), nasal and/or oral airflow via thermistor or pneumotachograph, oxygen saturation via pulse oximetry, body position, limb movements, recording of vibration, and end-tidal CO_2.[2]

5. Prior to the test, Mr. Apner should avoid stimulants, wear comfortable clothing (appropriate), and be sure to report at the correct time and place. Clients should be reminded of the contact phone number and be encouraged to call if they have questions.

6. Polysomnographic findings representing the presence of sleep apnea syndrome include "the presence of multiple obstructive or mixed apneas during sleep associated with repetitive episodes of inordinately loud snoring and excessive daytime sleepiness."[3] This is confirmed by polysomnographic representation of absence of or minimal presence of airflow in the presence of continued respiratory efforts. These data are analyzed and combined with the personal history, and diagnosis is made.

7. Laboratory data analysis:

   Hgb= 24 g/100 mL (elevated)
   ABG (represents chronic respiratory acidosis)

   These data indicate that Mr. Apner's pulmonary problems are longstanding. The hemoglobin level represents polycythemia (an elevated red cell mass), and the ABG represents chronic alveolar hypoventilation. These conditions are not likely to be effected by therapeutic interventions and should not be targeted as areas to improve (change). This is baseline data.

8. Potential problems associated with studying this patient in the sleep laboratory include skin irritation from adhesives used to apply various leads, physiologic reaction to adhesive remover at the study's end, electrical hazard, and eye irritation from adhesive.[4] General considerations addressing emergency and safety issues are also areas for concern.

9. Essential quality assurance tasks involving polysomnographic equipment include maintenance, calibration, verification of operation, upgrade, and repair of all equipment at appropriately scheduled time intervals, in accordance with recommendations and standards of manufacturers, the American Sleep Disorders Association (ASDA). The polysomnography guideline from the American Association for Respiratory Care also serves as an excellent source of information. A program to monitor and document the aforementioned, as well as ongoing auditing, are essential to maintenance of quality and improvement. The system used for these tasks must be organized so as to promote continuous compliance between and within all users of the polysomnographic equipment.

Because of the variety and complexity of the equipment used in this situation, precise checklists for per shift monitoring and checking of equipment is essential. All procedures and policies should be accessible at all times and written in such a manner so that communication is clear and orderly. Special attention should focus on any unexpected events, negative patient experiences, and technologist recommendations in order to provide continuous quality service. Assessment of the general environment is also essential. Needless to say, complete and accessible emergency supplies must be on hand at all times. They must be ready to use as well. All of the preceding tasks must be documented and verified according to policy.

10. OSAS.

11. Further study to determine appropriate intervention may be needed. CPAP levels can be titrated during the sleep study in order to determine the therapeutic level of CPAP. If NIPPV (noninvasive positive pressure ventilation of the Bi-PAP type) were chosen as treatment, levels of inspiratory and expiratory pressure could be titrated in the same manner.

12. Available treatments for obstructive sleep apnea syndrome include:[5]
    Oxygen
    Protriptyline
    Medroxyprogesterone
    Weight reduction
    Avoidance of Supine Sleeping Position
    Tongue retaining devices
    Nasopharyngeal airway
    Nasal continuous positive airway pressure (CPAP)
    Bi-level positive airway pressure
    Nasal surgery
    Tonsillectomy and adenoidectomy
    Uvulopalatopharyngoplasy
    Tracheostomy
    Mandibular, maxillary, and hyoid bone reconstruction

13. CPAP (continuous positive airway pressure) is commonly used in OSAS.

14. Example of RC plan:

    Indication: OSAS Intervention: CPAP at appropriate pressure level
    Objectives: Decrease incidence of apneas and associated symptoms
    Evaluation: Patient interview, follow-up sleep study

15. Instructions for home nasal CPAP.[7]

    Equipment preparation:

    1. Place blower unit on a level surface (table or nightstand) near where you sleep
    2. Make sure that the air exhaust and inlet vents are not obstructed
    3. Plug machine into a standard grounded (3-prong) electrical outlet

4. Check air inlet filter to be sure it is in place and free of dust
5. Connect one end of the tubing to the airflow outlet on the blower
6. Connect the other end of the tubing to the mask, then place the mask over the nose
7. Adjust strap tightness to seat mask firmly over nose
8. Turn on the blower and verify a flow of air
9. Assure proper fit and adjustment of mask and headgear. Air should not be leaking out around the bridge of the nose into the eyes.
10. You are now ready to sleep with mask on.

In the morning:

1. Remove mask by slipping strap off of back of head
2. Turn off blower
3. Wash the mask every morning with a mild detergent, then rinse with water. This keeps the mask soft and airtight.
4. Store the mask in plastic bag to keep free of dust and dirt

Weekly:

1. Wipe off the blower unit with a clean, damp cloth
2. Wash the headstrap
3. Service the filters according to the instructions in your patient manual

16. Mask fit is essential to successful therapy. The mask must be sized correctly so as not to be too small or large. Standard facial/nasal mask fitting devices are available for sizing a mask. Masks should fit securely and comfortably so as to negate leaks, assure equipment function, and remain in place but not so tightly that patient injury could occur.

Patient assessment should include a complete systematic evaluation of the patient during use of the CPAP system to assure proper function and safety.

Head straps must be adjusted to maintain mask fit and position. Leaks are particularly troublesome and common and therefore must be prevented and/or stopped. It is helpful to place the mask on the bridge of the nose and then adjust both sides of the headgear simultaneously.

17. This is a self-evaluation question.

18. Problems that may present in similar fashion to OSAS include:[9]

Narcolepsy
Insomnia
Hypometabolic states such a hypothermia, hypothyroidism
Uremia and other metabolic derangements
Cerebral vascular disease or other CNS degenerative disorders
Mental depression and other functional states
Sedatives or medications with sedating side-effects

19. Weight reduction combined with habituating nonsupine sleep position could have a beneficial effect over the long-term interval. The use of CPAP may be discontinued when symptoms subside.

20. Indications: OSAS Intervention: CPAP @ 12 cmH$_2$0

Objectives: reduce incidence of apneas, reduce symptoms of OSAS (hypersomnolence, snoring, etc.)

Evaluations: patient interview, physical assessment, follow-up study if needed

21. A change in the RC plan would be advised when patient improvement is noted, by achievement of objectives or when an adverse or unexpected response to treatment occurs. Examples of plan change indicators would be: patient refusal to comply with prescription, noncompliance due to patient intoler-

ance, worsening of general condition, or occurrence of negative physiologic responses such as an increase in dysrhythmias. Also if there is a lack of positive response to therapy the plan should be changed.

22. The RC plan should be evaluated on a timely basis (weekly, monthly, tri-monthly) in response to Mr. Apner's condition. As objectives are achieved the RC interventions should be discontinued.

23. See treatment algorithm (Figure 10-2 and 10-3).

References
1. Fletcher, E: Abnormalities of respiration during sleep. Grune & Stratton, Orlando, 1986, p. 13.
2. AARC Clinical Practice Guideline: Polysomnography. Respiratory Care, Dec. 1995, Vol. 40, no. 12, p. 1336.
3. Fletcher, et al. p. 13.
4. AARC et al. p. 1337.
5. Martin, R: Medical Treatment for the Sleep Apnea Syndrome. In: Fletcher, et al, p. 95.
6. Hudgel, D: Clinical Manifestations of the Sleep Apnea Syndrome. In: Fletcher, et al, p. 23.
7. Scanlan, C: Egan's Fundamentals of Respiratory Care. Mosby, 1995, p. 1125.

EXPERT OPINIONS FOR CHAPTER 11

1. In general, the patient's condition is good. Although her temperature is mildly elevated, she presents with normal heart and respiratory rate. Chest examination is negative for pulmonary infection or other disease process. Pulmonary mechanics are within normal ranges for this patient. Vital capacity is, however, on the low end of the spectrum. ABGs are good. Social history and current presentation are favorable in general, with no serious conditions or burdens being evident.

2. Mechanics of ventilation at this point in time are adequate. All test data indicate levels of ventilation above minimum acceptable levels.

3.
Interventions	Rationale
Monitoring via pulmonary mechanics	- to evaluate ventilatory status, detect problems
Performing ABGs	- to evaluate ventilatory and oxygenation status, detect problems
Cardiopulmonary assessment	- to evaluate aeration of lungs, integrity of thorax, and cardiac status
Evaluating plan	- to promote regulation of the plan in accordance with patient condition

4. Any parameters outside of the norm that might be detected that would indicate closer scrutiny or that would indicate possible need for increasing intervention.

5.
Indications	Objectives
Presence of Guillain Barre syndrome	- assess level of pulmonary deterioration - early detection of airway, ventilatory, or oxygenation problems

Interventions	Expected Outcomes
Perform mechanics	- detect problems of ventilation as they occur - detect diaphragmatic and accessory muscle paralysis - provide required RC services as needed
Perform ABGs	- detection of ventilation and oxygenation compromise as it occurs
Perform cardiopulmonary assessment q4 hr. Auscultation Percussion Inspection Palpation Vital signs	- detect signs of decreased aeration - detect changes in cardiac status - detect signs of infection - provide early interventions as indicated - detect airway compromise

6. This syndrome has acquired several names over the time span that it has been investigated. These include:[1]
   - infectious polyneuritis
   - acute idiopathic polyneuritis
   - Landry-Guillain-Barre-Stohl syndrome
   - Landry's paralysis
   - acute polyneuropathy
   - acute polyradiculitis
   - polyradiculoneuropathy

7. The patient's condition by 8:00AM on day 2 of admission reflects an improvement from her previously poor status. However, there is still a clear and present risk of ventilatory failure posed. This is manifested in the low values for mechanics. This patient may certainly begin a downward trend, necessitating intubation and PPV.

8. The indications for increasing the monitoring frequency are the poor mechanics, the increased heart rate, and the dropping PaO_2.

9. IPPB is indicated by the appearance of atelectasis combined with the need for ventilatory assistance, as evidenced by the drop in mechanics values. CPT is indicated by the atelectatic condition as well as the diminished VC, indicating lack of adequate cough mechanism.[3,4]

10. The objective of IPPB in this case is to improve CXR, improve breath sounds, and promote secretion clearance. The objective of CPT is to mobilize secretions to improve CXR, breath sounds, and clearance. [3,4]

11. Potential positive responses to IPPB in this case would include patient stability during treatment and fulfillment of the objectives as an outcome.

12. These two bronchial hygiene treatments will be stopped when the objectives of improvement in CXR, breath sounds, and secretion clearance are achieved.

13. If this patient continues to progress, her mechanics will improve, then plateau. She will possess a negative CXR, as well as clear breath sounds and cough. Her ABGs and vital signs will be adequate and she will not have respiratory distress. Her paralysis will cease and she will resume normal activities. If this patient continues to regress, her mechanics will worsen, indicating the need for intubation and PPV. Her paralysis could extend and respiratory failure may ensue. Worsening status may be identified by blood gas analysis, cardiopulmonary diagnostics, radiographic imaging, clinical observation, and physical examination, including vital signs.

14. Yes, it is entirely possible that the lateness of the RCP had an impact. The 2-hour delay (the schedule of monitoring called for checks every 4 hours) may have allowed patient care to be delivered at a less than optimal time. Earlier observations may have picked up on signs of worsening status and prompted earlier intervention.

15. Solutions for the RCP in a large facility with other staff members present would certainly include the delegation of either task to another staff member. A simple telephone call made from the emergency department (preferably placed by someone not involved in the emergency) could alert another staff member as to the problem at hand. Prioritizing would be essential. Solutions for the RCP working alone would not be as concise. The RCP could place a phone call to the ICU primary nurse for this patient and request the he or she perform careful cardiopulmonary assessments in the absence. Suggestions concerning what to look for might be helpful for the RCP to make to the nurse. Leaving the phone extension of the emergency department may also be helpful. Another possibility exists in delegating the emergency intubation assistance to other personnel capable of the responsibility, such as a medical resident, other physician, or nurse skilled in the area. In both cases it would be wise to alert the attending physician or perhaps a nursing supervisor of the dilemma. Other possible solutions may be afforded this way.

16. It is possible that the paralysis is reversing. Data supporting this assumption include the increase in vital capacity and maximum inspiratory pressure, as well as the improvement in oxygen saturation. Vital signs have also stabilized at acceptable values.

18. Hazards associated with IPPB include "increased airway resistance, barotrauma, nosocomial infection, hypocarbia, hemoptysis, hyperoxia when oxygen is the source gas, gastric distension, impaction of secretions, psychological dependence, impedance of venous return, exacerbation of hypoxemia, hypoventilation, increased mismatch of ventilation and perfusion, and air trapping."[4]

19. A decrease in venous return could be assessed in this case by a decrease in blood pressure or a change in pulse rate (the pulse may either increase or decrease in response to a drop in venous return, depending on how great a change occurs). Patient color may also change as venous return drops. Mottling, cyanosis or paleness may be seen. Physical signs may include diaphoresis and/or patient complaints. Changes in mentation may also occur.

20. Directed coughing is the teaching, supervising, and monitoring of techniques to mimic spontaneous coughing, when the latter is not present. The essential components of teaching the technique are preparation, instruction, demonstration, and evaluation. In preparing to teach directed coughing, one must understand the variety of available techniques, know the patient and history, and adapt the appropriate technique to the present situation. Instruction should include the description of what a cough is. This should include explaining that effective coughs incorporate deep inhalation (maximal inspiration), closure of the glottis (a breath hold), followed by a forceful exhalation (a strong cough out). Some circumstances may require that the RCP use manual assistance by applying pressure (usually with the hands) over the epigastric region to assist the exhalation. One other method may include the forced expiratory technique (huff coughing), which incorporates forceful "huffing" to aid in secretion mobilization. After explaining the procedure, the RCP should simply demonstrate the technique so that the learner may see it done. The demonstration may serve as a stimulus for questions as well. Lastly, the RCP should allow the patient to demonstrate the technique to assure proper usage. Evaluation should be performed in a caring and positive manner, assuring the patient as he or she practices in a nonthreatening and safe environment.[2]

21. PEP therapy certainly could have been used in this case. The advantages of using IPPB in this case include the improvement of aeration and assistance to ventilation that are available with the technique. PEP alone may only aid in secretion mobilization.

22. Individual maps will demonstrate the illustrator's unique perspectives and talents. Essential components of such concept maps should include allusion to improving pulmonary mechanics, vital signs, and physical examination. Patient progress to normal (pre-disease) status should be highlighted.

23. The RC plan at 6:00 PM on day 2 of hospitalization:

Indications	Objectives
- Presence of Guillain Barre syndrome	- Assess level of pulmonary involvement - Early detection of airway, ventilatory, or oxygenation problems

Interventions	Expected Outcomes
- Continue pulmonary mechanics q2 hr. - Continue IPPB with NaCl q2 hr.	- Evaluate ventilatory status, detect problems - Improved lung expansion - Mobilized secretions - Improved CXR
- Adjunct IPPB with directed coughing	- Improved secretion clearance - Promote self-care
- Perform ABG PRN - Continue cardiopulmonary assessment q 2 hr	- Detect problems of oxygenation and/or ventilation - Detect decreased aeration - Detect changes in cardiac status - Detect signs of infection - Provide early interventions, as indicated - Detect airway compromise
- Regulate plan	- Assess changes in status

References
1. DesJardins, T: Clinical Manifestations of Respiratory Disease, ed 2. Mosby, 1990, p 272.

2. AARC clinical practice guideline: Directed cough. Respiratory Care 38(5): 495, 1993.

3. AARC clinical practice guideline: Postural drainage therapy. Respiratory Care 36(12):1418, 1991.

4. AARC clinical practice guideline: Intermittent positive pressure breathing. Respiratory Care 38(11):1189, 1993.

5. AARC clinical practice guideline: Use of positive airway pressure adjuncts to bronchial hygiene therapy. Respiratory Care, 38(5):516, 1993.

6. Farzan, S: A Concise Handbook of Respiratory Disease, ed 3. Appleton-Lange, CT, 1992, p 315.

EXPERT OPINIONS FOR CHAPTER 12

1. The assessments made in the emergency room that indicate LTB as the problem are the presence of a barking cough, inspiratory and expiratory stridor, chest retractions, the history of an upper-respiratory infection, obvious respiratory distress, tachypnea, tachycardia, an oxygen saturation of 92%, and a radiograph revealing subglottic edema. The importance of the patient history as revealed by the parent is key in this case.

2. Examples of therapeutic objectives and expected outcomes related to the use of racemic epinephrine may include:

Objectives	Outcomes
- Decrease airway edema	- Stridor decreases/ceases
- Relieve airway obstruction	- Breathing pattern improves/normalizes
- Promote vasoconstriction of the airway	- Retractions subside
- Facilitate airway patency	- Radiograph (neck) improves
	- Cough dissipates
- Assure/improve oxygenation/ventilation	- Arterial blood gases improve
	- (Related to the above outcomes)
	- Absence of tachycardia
	- Related indices of oxygenation and ventilation improve
	- Pulmonary mechanics improve

3. Epiglottitis is mentioned in the case to draw attention to the need to differentiate between problems that present with similarities. The expectancy for students is that they will compare and contrast the problems of LTB, epiglottitis, and other upper-airway disorders. (The reference section of this chapter provides several good sources of information on the disorders.)

4. The assessments that indicate urgent need in this case would include all of the initial assessments mentioned previously (#1). It is particularly important to note the additive nature of these data, as some information in itself is not indicative of urgency. When viewed together, the data clearly indicate that urgency exists. The concept of preventing further patient deterioration is worthy of discussion at this point. Also, examination of the practitioner's feelings in such a case, as well as consideration for the child and parents, creates an opportunity to integrate the concepts of coping with crisis, empathy, and professional communication into the case.

5. A flow diagram representing an assess and treat protocol may look as follows:

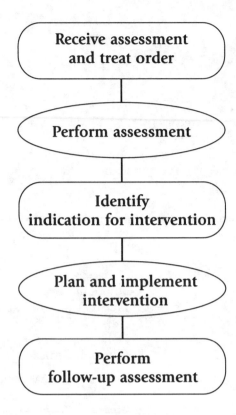

6. A safety checklist/policy for the use of mist tents should include the following points of interest:
    - Posting of No Smoking signs
    - Advisement to parents, child, and staff that no friction-producing objects be allowed inside the tent (computer games, televisions, music boxes, nurse calls, etc.)
    - Observation of correct tent assembly:
        - Appropriate aerosol delivery and flow
        - Analysis of oxygen percentage in use
        - Compliance with prescription
        - Canopy tucked under mattress
        - Zipper openings appropriate to maintenance of FiO_2
    - Environmental temperature is assessed as practical
    - Patient is positioned comfortably inside tent and is assured of safety
    - Parent involvement and education is fostered
    - Equipment safety and cleanliness are assured
    - Therapeutic plan is complete and documentation is assured

    Combining this listing/mapping activity with actual tent assemble (in a laboratory or practice environment) may foster deeper learning.

7. The AARC CPG on bland aerosol administration[1] lists the following:

Indications	Assessment of Need	Assessment of Outcome
Upper airway edema	Presence of:	Decreased work of breathing
Bypassed airway	stridor	Improved vital signs
Sputum induction	brassy, croupy cough	Decreased stridor
	hoarseness after extubation	Decreased dyspnea
	diagnosis of LTB or croup	Improved ABG

clinical history suggesting	Improved oximetry values
upper airway irritation	Adequate sputum production for sampling
increased work of breathing	(induction achieved)
(i.e., smoke inhalation)	
need for sputum induction	

Analysis of this information presents a representation of three basic problems, their related assessment data, and outcomes to be achieved in their treatment. The three basic problems are notably upper-airway edema, airway bypass via intubation, and the need for sputum induction. Integrating the CPG into case study work lends clarity and validity to the students' practice.

8. Intubation in this case is indicated by the summing of several factors. Arterial blood gases indicate respiratory failure with hypoxemia. Physical signs include cyanosis and increased work of breathing with retractions and flaring. Signs of physical exhaustion and inability to maintain ventilation are present including a decrease in respiratory rate from 32–15; an increase in heart rate from 140–160 with subsequent drop in blood pressure and palpation of thready pulse; and a decrease in level of consciousness. Discussion of the significance and cause of these changes may promote both interest and anxiety in students. It seems prudent to allow time for investigation, integration, and incubation of these physiologic findings. Further learning activities might include data papers, concept mapping of the individual problems (i.e., cardiovascular anatomy and physiology, airway anatomy, causes of hypoxemia, ventilation review, diagramming of similar cases.)

9. The missing information for figure 12-1:[2]

Defining Characteristics	Pathophysiology	Interventions
Age: 6 mo–3 yr	Area of edema: larynx, trachea, bronchi	O2 delivery: mist tent with O_2
Auscultation findings: stridor	Etiology: viral	Medications: racemic epinephrine
Radiologic findings: narrowing of subglottic region often referred to as the steeple sign	Effect on airway resistance: increases	Fluids
	Effect on oxygenation: deteriorates	Comfort/safety:
	Effect on ventilation: deteriorates	- maintain cool mist
		- follow safety checklist for equipment setup
		- maintain adequate communication
		- promote parental involvement and education

10. Pat Garcia's RC plan: @ 10:20 PM on day 1.

Assessment of indications for RC:
   - Diagnosis of laryngotracheobronchitis in a 2-year-old child
   - Deterioration in oxygen status
   - Ventilatory failure determined by arterial blood gas
   - Decreased sensorium
   - Artificial airway in place: #4.0 cuffless oral endotracheal tube

Interventions indicated:
   - Perform airway care/suctioning PRN
   - Institute mechanical ventilation:
      SIMV
      f=10
      Vt= 60 mL

FiO_2 = .50
Vpeak= 18 L/min
PEEP= 5 cmH_2O
alarms set as follows:
    High inspiratory pressure = 15cm H_2O > Pawp
    Low inspiratory pressure = 10 cm H_2O < Pawp
    Low tidal volume = 45 mL
    Low FiO_2 = .45
    High FiO_2 = .55
    Low PEEP = 3 cm H_2O
apnea (back-up) parameters functional
- wean via decreasing respiratory rate and decreasing FiO_2
- provide educational service to parents

Therapeutic objectives:
- Maintain airway patency
- Extubate when airway edema decreases to the point where an audible leak can be heard around
  endotracheal tube at peak airway pressure
- Maintain PaO_2 > 80 mmHg to assure oxygenation
- Maintain $PaCO_2$ between 35 and 45 to assure ventilation
- Maintain pH between 7.35 and 7.45 to assure acid-base balance
- Provide 100% relative humidity via heated humidifier
- Perform operational verification procedure prior to placing patient on ventilator
- Verify operation of ventilator alarms and limits
- Maintain airway temperature at 37°C
- Perform system checks every 2 hours or after changes are made to assure safety and function
- Maintain compliance with physician orders
- Monitor FDO_2 when changes are made or at least every 24 hr.
- Wean from MV while maintaining previous objectives
- Identify and correct patient problems associated with treatment
- Document findings on an ongoing basis
- Facilitate parental understanding and comfort

Evaluations to be performed:
- Arterial blood gas analysis after ventilator or status changes
- Continuous pulse oximetry
- Continuous electrocardiography
- Monitor vital signs
- Auscultate chest and neck
- Perform pulmonary assessments via observation, palpation, and percussion
- Monitor radiographs, evaluate airway edema and general chest appearance
- Monitor and evaluate peak airway pressure, spontaneous ventilatory data, plateau pressures, alarm
  occurrences, and all other data from ventilatory/patient system checks
- Evaluate sputum production
- Monitor and evaluate pulmonary mechanics
- Monitor lab data and other significant data
- Evaluate and record patient progress notations including overall status report
- Assess parental level of understanding regarding child's condition

Expected outcomes:
- Dyspnea will cease
- Secretions will be managed
- Parents and child will demonstrate less anxiety over the condition
- Parents will vocalize their level of understanding the disease process, as well as the expected outcome

11. The decrease in FiO_2 from .50 to .40 is indicated at this time. The oxygen indices that are available
    (PaO_2 and SaO_2) reveal oxygenation in excess of normal values. A 10% decrease is indicated in light of
    the excessive PaO_2 of 200 mmHg.

12. A checklist for in-hospital patient-ventilator transport should include:[3]
    - Operational verification of transport ventilator
    - Verification of function and duration of oxygen and air cylinders
    - Ventilator system check before and after transport
    - Presence and function of monitors:
       ECG, oximetry, hemodynamic monitors (at least blood pressure monitoring equipment), carbon dioxide detectors, stethoscope, oxygen analyzer
    - Medication/fluid checklist
    - Documentation record

13. The decision to remove the endotracheal tube from the child's mouth was sound. Evidence citing visualization of a kink in the tube is noted to support the decision. The patient also demonstrated signs of severe respiratory distress. The choice to reintubate was a sound one.

14. The incident occurred just after a transport situation. A number of hazards exist during transport, one of which is dislodging of the artificial airway. The hazards are related to the movement of the patient and the many pieces of apparatus that are transported. It is likely in this case that the airway became dislodged at or after admission to the PICU, as there is a clinical notation stating that the patient was stable during the transport.

15. A smaller endotracheal tube was required during the second intubation because of further airway edema. Most likely the cause of this condition was the irritation from being intubated.

16. The significance of having "no leak" when the ETT was placed is that this indicates a very "tight" fit. This presents a risk of increasing the airway edema, related to tissue injury. However, improvement in the airway condition may be easily assessed when a leak is noted.

17. Considering that LTB is commonly of viral origin it is probable that the airway edema will subside when the virus has "run its course." In such a case intubation may be required for about 48–72 hours.

18. Indications for extubation in this case would be:
    - Audible leak around ETT at peak airway pressure of 20–30 cm H_2O.
    - Pulmonary mechanics indicate adequate ventilation
    - Arterial blood gases are within normal ranges
    - The patient is awake and alert
    - Spontaneous ventilatory parameters are adequate
    - Secretions are minimal
    - No signs of respiratory distress are present

19: A postextubation RC plan for Pat Garcia may include:

Objectives	- Maintain/improve airway patency - Monitor and evaluate signs of increase in airway resistance - Maintain/improve oxygenation and ventilation - Mobilize secretions - Improve breath sounds
Interventions	- Aerosolized racemic epinephrine postextubation and PRN following (via small volume nebulizer) - Provide cool humidity via mist tent powered by compressed air—continuously - Promote deep breathing and coughing every hour - Identify and correct problems that occur
Evaluations	- Monitor breath sounds for the presence of stridor or other adventitious sounds - Check vital signs before and after treatment - Monitor and interpret ECG

- Pulse oximetry continuous
- Measure vital capacity, tidal volume, and maximal inspiratory pressure q 4 hr for 24 hr.
- Monitor breathing pattern and general appearance
- Medical record review and documentation on an ongoing basis

Expected Outcomes
- Child resumes normal activity
- Dyspnea and cough cease
- Parents demonstrate knowledge of early warning signs of LTB and indicate appropriate interventions (i.e., when to seek help)

20. Examples of upper airway conditions that present in a similar fashion to LTB include epiglottitis, other croup syndromes, and foreign body aspiration.

21.

Condition	Similarities to LTB	Differences from LTB[2,4]
Epiglottitis	Stridor may be present Respiratory distress may be present	Bacterial in origin (H-influenza) Area of edema is the epiglottis Lateral neck radiograph reveals swollen epiglottis but not the steeple sign of LTB
Foreign body aspiration	Stridor may be present Respiratory distress may be present	History of aspirating or swallowing object Radiograph may reveal the object

Patients being treated for epiglottitis will receive antibiotic therapy. Racemic epinephrine would not provide effective vasoconstriction to manage the swollen epiglottis. Patients being treated for foreign body aspiration would most likely undergo therapeutic bronchoscopy for removal of the object. (Abdominal thrusts may be indicated as well.) Again, the standard treatments for LTB would not be effective for foreign body aspiration. These represent only two upper-airway problems. Numerous others exist and may be classified into infectious, congenital, or acquired problems.

References

1. AARC clinical practice guidelines: Bland aerosol administration. Respiratory Care 38(11):1196,1993.
2. Whitaker, K: Comprehensive Perinatal and Pediatric Respiratory Care. Delmar, NY, 1992, p. 452.
3. AARC clinical practice guidelines: Transport of the mechanically ventilated patient. Respiratory Care 38(11):1169, 1993.
4. Thompson, JE, Farrell, E, and McManus M: Neonatal and pediatric airway emergencies. Respiratory Care 37(6):582, 1992.

EXPERT OPINIONS FOR CHAPTER 13

Note: These answers are focused on the thinking process. Individual wording may differ widely. Student learners and experts alike may have significant additional information to add.

1. Indications for MV: apnea, postresuscitation condition:

Interventions	Objectives
Settings for MV:	-Improve oxygenation
Vt—650 mL	-Improve ventilation
RR 12	-Maintain airway
FiO_2 1.00	-Prevent lung injury (assoc. with PPV)
Vpeak 50 L/min	-Promote stable vital signs
PEEP 5 cm H_2O	

    Safe ranges for alarm settings:

Pressure	—High (10 cmH_2O > PIP)
	—Low (10 cmH_2O < PIP)
Oxygen	—High (100%)
	—Low (95%)
PEEP	—High (8 cmH_2O)
	—Low (3 cmH_2O)
Low exhaled volume (550 mL)	
Low exhaled VE (6.5 L/min)	
Maintain airway temperature (approx. 37°C)	

    Expected outcomes:

    - Oxygenation and ventilation will be adequate
    - CXR will be clear
    - Secretions will be negligible
    - Patient will successfully wean from MV
    - No harmful effects of PPV will occur
    - Vital signs will remain stable

2. The recorded actions were appropriate.

3. Supplies needed for transport of this child include:[1,2]
    - Transport ventilator in full operational order
    - Hygroscopic condensor humidifier
    - All medications the patient is currently requiring
    - Resuscitation supplies (resuscitator, O_2 source, medications, airway management tools)
    - Infection control supplies (gloves, masks, gowns, etc.)
    - Clamps, scissors, forceps, surgical supplies (sutures etc.)
    - Portable lighting
    - First aid supplies
    - Blood gas equipment
    - Catheterization and collection equipment
    - Monitors (stethoscope, hand-held spirometer, stethoscope, pulse oximeter, ECG monitor, hemodynamic monitor, blood pressure cuff and doppler device, oxygen analyzer, laboratory equipment for collection of specimens, transcutaneous monitors, pressure manometer)

Safety procedures include:
- Operational verification of transport ventilator
- Verification of function and duration of oxygen and air cylinders
- Ventilator system check before and after transport
- Presence and function of monitors:
    ECG, oximetry, hemodynamic monitors (at least blood pressure monitoring equipment), carbon dioxide detectors, stethoscope, oxygen analyzer
- Medication/fluid checklist
- Documentation record

4. Hazards associated with air transport of this patient may include risks associated with airway obstruction, accidental extubation, equipment malfunction or breakage, IV line removal, injury to patient/staff from movement or fall, change in ventilation due to mechanical ventilation, changes in partial pressure of oxygen due to increasing altitude, and expansion of gases within the body related to increasing altitude.[2]

5. Since maintenance of PaO_2 under conditions of increased altitude will require increasing the delivered oxygen percentage, the RCP will need to monitor oxygenation by ABG, oximetry, or transcutaneous monitor in order to titrate the oxygen percentage during the flight.

6. Since this patient is hypothermic, all measures to consistently increase the core temperature must be maintained. Warming of the inspired air is one such measure.[3]

7. Measures used to rewarm a hypothermic victim include airway rewarming; heated IV solutions; heated lavage of the gastric, intrathoracic, pericardial, and peritoneal spaces and the urinary bladder and rectum; and extracorporeal circulation. External measures such as warming blankets, warm baths, and near-total immersion in a Hubbard tank have also been used. Use of these measures is dependent on the severity of the hypothermia and the availability of the resources.[3]

8 . The antibiotic preparation is given to prevent infection associated with the aspiration of water, residue from the pond, and/or gastric secretions.

9. When cooling of the body precedes an asphyxic episode, survival is possible for near-drowning victims. Survival after as long as 1 hour has been recorded. The hypothermic state is protective to the human organism in many ways. Most are related to the general depression of metabolic function initiated by the hypothermia.[4]

10. The ABG recorded at 5:30PM represents respiratory and metabolic acidosis with severe hypoxemia.

11. In calculating the tank duration of a full "E" cylinder running at 5 L/min, one finds the following:

    (tank factor) .28 $\times$ (tank pressure) 2000 = 12 min. or 1 hr., 52 min liter flow)[5]

    Although 1 hour and 52 minutes allows enough gas for the supposed 33-minute flight, one must assure that a back-up source (most likely a compressed gas cylinder) is present. This safety procedure will decrease the risks associated with unaccounted for delays in transport as well as unexpected equipment problems. Therefore, although one cylinder will suffice for the gas supply, a back-up source is essential.

12. The neurologic status of the patient, that is, being comatose and unresponsive, is clearly poor. The condition may have several contributing causes. It is likely that hypoxemia, hypothermia, asphyxia, and aspiration have contributed to the problem. It is also possible that other underlying problems may exist. Traumatic injuries, airway obstruction, organ failure, diffuse intravascular coagulation, and infectious processes should not be overlooked.[3]

13. A score of 4 on the Glasgow Coma Scale indicates a deep coma revealing little response to stimuli. (See Appendix D, "Glasgow Coma Scale.")

14. The maximum rating that can be generated using the Glasgow Coma Scale is a value of 15 points, indicating an individual who is able to spontaneously open the eyes, obey verbal commands, and express appropriate orientation by verbal response.

15. Other than the comatose state, the pupils are not reacting and are dilated. Also, the presence of apnea indicates poor neurological function.

16. It is quite possible that the neurologic effects of the submersion incident are temporary.[3,4,5]

17. RC objectives:
    - Maintain oxygenation (maintain PaO_2 > 55)
    - Maintain ventilation (maintain $PaCO_2$ between 35 and 45 with pH between 7.35 and 7.45)
    - Maintain patent airway
    - Improve aeration, prevent progression of pulmonary infection and congestion
    - Improve CXR
    - Improve breath sounds
    - Increase core temperature to 37° C
    - Maintain stable vital signs
    - Minimize mechanical inflation pressures
    - Prevent equipment malfunctions

18. The objective for bronchial hygiene treatment of this patient is to prevent progression of an infectious pneumonia related to aspiration.

19. Indications for increasing the PEEP level at 7:30PM on day 1 include PaO_2 of 68 on FiO_2 of 1.00 and with 5 cmH_2O of PEEP; a Pa-etCO$_2$ gradient of 14 torr; an AaO_2 gradient of 615; and an estimated shunt (Qs/Qt) of 22%. Each of these factors is associated with the need to increase the level of PEEP.[6,7]

20. Positive responses to PPV would include improvements in oxygenation and ventilation; occurrence of spontaneous movements (e.g., respirations); stable vital signs; increase in core temperature; improvement in hemodynamic values; improvement in CXR (clearing); improvement in sputum consistency and reduction in production; and improvement in chest examination (breath sounds, percussion notes, skin color, etc.).

21. Negative responses to PPV may be assessed by lack of improvement in the areas stated in question 17 and 21, as well as by increases in peak airway pressures signaling worsening chest compliance (a decrease in CLst) or airway resistance (an increasing Raw), lung injury; or by signs of cardiovascular embarrassment, renal compromise, or cerebral insult.[8]

22. The pulmonary status of this patient at this point in time indicates that a problem associated with low static lung compliance (Clst = 14mL/cm/H_2O), high pulmonary artery pressure (45/30 torr), high pulmonary capillary wedge pressure (31 torr), and a large shunt fraction (22%), exists. This would reflect cardiogenic pulmonary edema in essence. However, in this case the data reflect the overriding diagnosis of near drowning, which includes the problem of pulmonary edema within it.[5]

23. Should this patient deteriorate further, there are several techniques that may be of use. These include pressure-controlled ventilation, inverse ratio ventilation (pressure or volume oriented), high-frequency ventilation, and extracorporeal membrane oxygenation. Interventions such as permissive hypercapnia and surfactant therapy have shown promise in the treatment of ARDS and thus hold potential in the treatment of a near-drowning victim, requiring PPV with high inflation pressures, hypoxemia, and low static compliance, as well.[9,10]

24. The hemodynamic data generated on this first clinical day for Meg Swimm (PAP, PCWP) describe a condition that produces increased pressure in the pulmonary system (PAP) and the left heart (PCWP). This would generally be termed cardiogenic pulmonary edema. The contributing factors in this case

are the aspiration of fluid and gastric material as well as the global hypothermic vasoconstriction and capillary injury. In considering that the PCWP is increased it must also be assumed that there is a left heart problem. This may be related to the hypothermia, asphyxia, and aspiration as well.[11]

25. FiO_2 was cautiously weaned from 1.00 to .85 by 10:00PM. Prior to this decrease in FiO_2 was an increase in the PEEP level. Indicators of adequate oxygenation in this case include PaO_2, AaO_2, PvO_2, So_2, CaO_2, and Qs/Qt. PEEP was increased to the point where oxygenation and pulmonary compliance were maximized, while blood pressure and cardiac output were optimal. Once an appropriate PEEP level was secured the FiO_2 was lowered and the response was assessed.

26. At this point in the case it is time to refocus and readjust the RC plan. Current objectives might emphasize a structured weaning approach, prevention of lung injury from PPV, and early discharge planning. (Although it may seem premature to plan for the discharge of this patient, it is in fact never too early. In projecting the course of progress in such a case one may assume that a great deal of intervention accompanied by a lengthy hospital stay is inevitable. To minimize these conditions, early discharge planning inclusive of parental involvement is key. Obviously a team approach to this part of the plan is essential.)[12]

27. An increasing time span between evaluations of the plan will most likely be in order here. For instance the critical care part of this plan should be evaluated approximately every 24–48 hours. The next phase of the plan occurring after transfer to a "step-down" unit could be evaluated every 72–168 hours. As the patient progresses to subacute care of some type, the plan's evaluation would occur less often, perhaps initially weekly to monthly, then progressively to 3-month periods. As long as this patient was receiving respiratory care it is likely that the 3- month period of evaluation would remain fixed, as a verification of need, progress, and care.

28. Discharge RC plan:

Objectives	Interventions
A. - Meg Swimm will remain free of pulmonary infection	- airway care - circuit changes - system checks - bronchial hygiene
B. - M.S. will maintain adequate oxygenation and ventilation	- PPV - monitoring (ABG, oximetry, physical exam, pulmonary mechanics)
C. - Weaning from PPV will be promoted	- use of pressure support—continue IMV use - physical conditioning (team objective)/ with RC focus on deep breathing

D.- M.S.'s parents will demonstrate:
  - emergency care techniques (CPR)
  - ability to perform routine care of mechanical ventilator
  - knowledge of equipment and its function
  - assessment skill regarding signs of pulmonary distress/ infection/airway obstruction
  - appropriate suctioning, CPT, manual resuscitation, and airway care procedures
  - correct administration technique of medications[13]
	- education and evaluation

Expected outcomes:

- The achievement of the objectives listed

- Evaluations will be performed on a timely and planned basis

29. Refer to objective "D" above.

References

1. Whitaker, K: Comprehensive Perinatal and Pediatric Respiratory Care. Delmar, NY, 1992, p 611.
2. AARC clinical practice guidelines: Transport of the mechanically ventilated patient. Respiratory Care 38(11): 1169, 1993.
3. Nemiroff, MJ: Near Drowning. Respiratory Care 37(6): 600, 1993.
4. Nemiroff MJ, Saltz, GR, and Weg, JR: Survival after cold water near drownings: The protective effect of the diving reflex (abstract). Am Rev Resp Dis 115(4): 145, 1977.
5. Moore, GC: Near drowning. In Levin DL, Morriss, FC, and Moore, GC: A Practical Guide to Pediatric Intensive Care, ed 2. Mosby, St Louis, 1984, p 180.
6. Steinberg, KP and Pierson DJ: Clinical approach to the patient with acute oxygenation failure. In Pierson, DJ and Kacmarek RM: Foundations of Respiratory Care. Churchill Livingstone, NY, 1992, p 727.
7. Pierson DJ, Kacmarek RM: Positive end-expiratory pressure: State of the art after 29 years. Respiratory Care 33: 419, 1988.
8. Pilbeam, S: Mechanical Ventilation. Mosby, St Louis, 1991.
9. East, TD: The magic bullets in the war on ARDS: Aggressive therapy for oxygenation failure. Respiratory Care 38(6): 690, 1993.
10. Heulitt, MJ, Anders, M, and Benham, D: Acute respiratory distress syndrome in pediatric patients: Redirecting therapy to reduce iatrogenic lung injury. Respiratory Care 40(1): 74.
11. Farzan, S: A Concise Handbook of Respiratory Diseases, ed 3. Appleton and Lange, CT, 1992, p 268.
12. O'Ryan, J: Discharge planning for the respiratory patient. In Lucas, J, Golish, JA, Sleeper, G, and O'Ryan J: Home Respiratory Care. Appleton and Lange, CT, 1988, p 229.
13. Whitaker, K: Comprehensive Perinatal and Pediatric Respiratory Care. Delmar, NY, 1992, p 628.

EXPERT OPINIONS FOR CHAPTER 14

1. Immediate interventions include oxygen therapy (indicated by SpO_2), narcotics for pain, assurance of physical rest, and full continuous monitoring/assessment.

2. The ECG represents acute anterior transmural infarction.

3. Assessments supporting the diagnosis, aside from the ECG, are presence of chest pain, diaphoresis, dyspnea, tachycardia, tachypnea hypotension, nausea, and the history of the event.

4. Assessment plan: Patient's description of chest pain, vital signs, ECG, oximetry, sensorium, appearance, heart and breath sounds, breathing pattern, urine output, palpation of extremities (for coolness, moistness), serial enzymes, and ABG. These should be performed continuously or hourly.

5. Complications of myocardial infarction include dysrhythmias, pulmonary edema, shock, cardiac arrest, death, thrombosis, and myocardial trauma.

6. Additional risk factors listed include hypertension, history of bronchitis, smoking history, overweight status, and family history of cardiac disease.

7. Assessments supporting the diagnosis of MI are the description of the ECG, presence of chest pain, patient history, physical appearance, hypotension, and respiratory status.

8. The indications for intubation include respiratory failure with hypoxemia and presence of MI.

9. Appropriate ventilatory settings for MV (institutional policy should be consulted in actual cases):

Mode:	IMV
Vt:	800 mL
f:	12
FiO_2:	1.00
Vpeak:	60 L/min
PEEP:	5 cm H_2O

   Alarm settings and limits:
   Low Vt: 700 mL
   High f: 30 BPM
   Low inspiratory pressure: 10–15 cm below Pawp
   Low PEEP: 3 cm H_2O
   High inspiratory pressure: 10–15 cm H_2O > Pawp
   Low minute ventilation: 8.0 L/min
   Apnea settings: as per policy
   Low FiO_2: 95%

10. Objectives for the RC plan:
    1. Improve oxygenation
    2. Assure adequate ventilation
    3. Maintain tissue perfusion
    4. Maintain equipment/patient safety
    5. Promote patient comfort

11. Streptokinase is a thrombolytic agent. Negative effects associated with administration of this agent include systemic bleeding, dysrhythmias, allergic reactions, and recurrent thrombosis.

12. The hemodynamic data indicate that cardiogenic shock has occurred.

13. This problem is most likely a consequence of the MI.

14. The urine output of 12 mL/hr is very low and supports the diagnosis of cardiogenic shock.

15. Problems that may have been precipitated by MV include increased hypotension, tachycardia, decreased urine output, and the total picture of cardiogenic shock (see: hemodynamic data).

16. Transport of this critical patient would require:

Equipment	Precautions
Airway management supplies	Avoid hyperventilation when hand resuscitator is used
Self-inflating resuscitation bag	Monitor parameters for changes
Portable oxygen source	Avoid problems associated with position changes
Transport ventilator (if available)	Monitor ECG
Pulse oximeter	Maintain IV patency
ECG/vascular monitor	Assure quality of equipment and procedures
Pharmocologic agents required	Monitor all equipment connections especially ventilator
Stethoscope	tubing and airway patency
Hygroscopic condenser for humidity	Provide adequate gas and flow
Spirometer/manometer	

17. The primary goals of IABC are:

    1. Attain normal/adequate tissue perfusion
    2. Optimize hemodynamic function
    3. Prevent complications related to procedure
    4. Maintain patient safety/comfort

18. The RCP may participate in the roles of:

    -assisting the physician with preparation, insertion, and operation of the devices
    -monitoring the patient and equipment during and after use
    -providing postprocedure care
    -implementing quality assessments surrounding the procedure and equipment

19. Positive effects of therapy would include achieving the goals of the RC plan.

    1. Improve oxygenation
    2. Assure adequate ventilation and of the IABC intervention as well
    3. Attain normal/adequate tissue perfusion
    4. Optimize hemodynamic function
    5. Prevent complications related to procedure
    6. Maintain patient safety/comfort

20. Negative effects would include problems associated with complications of the interventions (MV, IABC medications) or progression of the patient's problem state (further cardiopulmonary sequelae).

21. The therapist depicted in the notations revealed sound resource management abilities by requesting assistance at the earliest sign of being involved in a nonroutine, time-consuming task (assisting with IABC initiation). This strategy will optimize patient care in general.

22. The three primary goals that must be achieved before successful discharge of this MI patient are:

    1. Attain normal/adequate tissue perfusion
    2. Optimize hemodynamic function
    3. Assure oxygenation/ventilation

23. The RC department may serve Mable Cash by providing assistance in smoking cessation and cardiac rehabilitation (health promotion).

24. Outcome criteria for this case may include:

    - Symptom management (reports symptoms of significance immediately)
    - Client makes activity modifications during recovery
    - Participates in rehabilitation program of activities (physical conditioning on an ongoing basis)

25. The psychological issues that may require attention include anxiety related to condition, fear of complications, depression, hopelessness, and noncompliance to the plan.

EXPERT OPINIONS FOR CHAPTER 15

1. The physical assessments are interpreted as follows:

Assessment	Interpretation
- Postoperative... with nocturnal NIPPV and continuous supplemental oxygen need	Represents poor pulmonary but due to the acuteness of the postsurgical condition, indicates good potential for rehabilitation.
- 76-yr-old man	An elderly man may have age-related issues. Analyze data with this special population in mind.
- Pale, thin	? nutritional status, ? RBC
- Dyspneic	Likely due to a combination of several problems; should be used as a guide during activity.
- Alert	Positive sign—a definite plus for following a rehabilitation plan.
- Depressed	Not unusual for someone in Mr. Babson's present condition; must be continually assessed and considered when care planning. Mr. Babson may require considerable positive reinforcement and encouragement. Psychological services may be needed.
- Decreased BS	A common finding in COPD
- Resonant percussion	Also common
- CXR:hyperaerartion	Also common (all represent hyperinflation)
- PFT (obstruction noted)	Typical of COPD... particularly common in emphysema
- Early desaturation when exercising	Supports need for oxygen therapy... can be used as baseline for goal setting in physical reconditioning
- Hct and Hgb	Represent polycythemia, (45%....19); common in chronic hypoxemia
- ABG: $PaO_2 = 65$ $PaCO_2 = 66$ pH = 7.36 $HCO_3 = 42$	Represents chronic alveolar hypoventilation with hypoxemia
- Vital signs: BP = 155/95	Mild hypertension
RR = 16	Normal
HR =106	Mild tachycardia

The primary problems identified are his postoperative condition combined with the history of COPD and subsequent oxygen dependence. The current need for nocturnal ventilatory assistance is also a primary problem.

2. Mr. Babson may be classified as being in "poor condition," as revealed by a score of 17 on the assessment scoring system presented. He is classified as having a score of "3" in all areas, except for scoring a "2" in "other organ system problems." Note the circled categories for Mr. Babson, below:

Assessments	GOOD CONDITION 1	FAIR CONDITION 2	POOR CONDITION 3
Ability to perform ADLs	Performs all self-care	Requires some assistance	Cannot perform
Level of dyspnea	No dyspnea	Dyspnea on exertion	Continual dyspnea
Duration of required supplemental O_2 use	None or only used with exercise	<12 hr/day	Continuous (nocturnal)
PFT	Mild disease	Moderate disease	Severe disease
Exercise testing	Tolerates 6 min of walking	Walks at least 3 min without desat.	Cannot perform
Other organ system	None	One other system	>1 other with problem

3. Short-term goal: increase activity tolerance
   Long-term goal: decrease supplemental oxygen use; decrease dependence on NIPPV.

4. The RC plan:

Indications	Objectives	Interventions	Outcome Evaluations
Low oxygen indices	Assure oxygenation	Oxygen therapy	ABG/pulse oximetry/vital signs
Respiratory insufficiency/unstable ventilatory drive	Assure ventilation	NIPPV	ABG/pulse oximetry/vital signs/level of dyspnea
COPD	Improve exercise tolerance/promote self-care/improve breathing pattern, efficiency/promote pulmonary hygiene	Initiate pulmonary rehabilitation	Activity tolerance/breathing pattern/exercise testing/follow-up questionnaire

5. Suggested settings for NIPPV:[1]

   Volume ventilation: or   Pressure support ventilation (BiPAP):
   Vt = 15–20 mL/Kg.   RR = 15–20
   RR = 15–20 BPM   EPAP = 5cm H_2O
   I:E = 1:1 to 1:3   IPAP = 15–22 (to adjust $PaCO_2$)

   supplemental oxygen as indicated

6. Essential components of a rehabilitation plan:

   Intake interviewing, communicating, planning
   Introduction/overview
   Pulmonary anatomy, physiology and pathology of disease
   Breathing techniques
   Relaxation, stress management
   Exercise and personal routine techniques
   Pulmonary hygiene techniques
   Administration of oxygen and aerosol therapy, other procedures
   Medications
   Recreation and vocational counseling
   Maintenance of conditioning
   Evaluation, follow-up

7. Suggested discharge plan:

Objectives
- optimize oxygenation/ventilation
- promote self-care
- improve exercise tolerance
- decrease symptom occurrence
- decrease technologic dependence

Interventions
- oxygen therapy (with exertion)
- NIPPV (nocturnal/PRN)
- pulmonary rehabilitation
- discharge to safe home environment
- promote compliance with plan
- educate patient and family
- facilitate relationship with home care agency

Outcomes
- improved ABG, oximetry, lab values
- less dyspnea (per observation and subjective statements)
- improved exercise tolerance (per walking oximetry testing)
- improved self-care abilities (per survey questionnaire and observation)

8. Discharge planning team members:[2]

Team Member	Duties
Physician	Does final assessment of patient, writes all drug and equipment prescriptions
Respiratory therapist	Evaluates all facets of patient's respiratory status, reviews equipment and supplies needs
Nurse	Assesses all bodily needs, individually and as a whole, and writes initial home care plan
Physical therapist	Evaluates patient's current musculoskeletal status, reviews all self-care patient must perform with self and family
Dietician	Writes home nutrition plan, makes sure patient will have adequate nutritive intake or makes alternate plan (e.g., Meals on Wheels)
Occupational therapist	Reassesses patient's gains since occupational therapy began in hospital and informs home care team of strengths and weaknesses
Psychiatrist/psychologist	Writes patient profile summary and shares allowable areas with home care team
Social worker	Checks and double-checks to make certain all outside agencies involved with patient's home care are ready to assist and have all red tape out of the way
Pastoral member	Makes arrangements to see patient on regular basis once patient is home or sees as needed

9. A breathing retraining program may focus on the teaching and learning of pursed lip breathing, diaphragmatic breathing, and relaxation techniques.

10. Liquid oxygen systems are detailed as follows:[3]

Advantages	Disadvantages
The system of choice for the continuous high-volume user	Oxygen waste and additional expense incurred as a result of evaporative losses if not used on a nearly continuous basis
Ability of active patient outside the home to fill his or her own portable system	Regular deliveries are required
No electrical operation	Personal injury may occur from handling of extremely cold transfilling fittings by patients or home care personnel

Large-volume capacity in small space
Capable of being used in a wide range of pressure
applications

11. Mr. Babson would use a portable liquid oxygen (LOX) system to ambulate and exercise with. This LOX portable should be filled as follows:[4]

1. Make sure there is enough liquid oxygen in the reservoir.
2. Check the connectors on both units to make sure that they are clean and dry. Moisture on these connectors could cause the connectors to freeze together.
3. Connect the portable unit to the reservoir according to the manufacturer's instructions. The flowrate controller should be turned off.
4. Open the portable unit vent. Allow the portable unit to fill until the vent begins to pass liquid oxygen instead of gas. Close the vent valve.
5. Disengage the portable unit according to the manufacturer's instructions.

As with any equipment assembly, all needed supplies (reservoir, portable tank, gloves for hands...) should be gathered first.

All safety precautions indicated when using oxygen should be observed. The unit should be checked for operation by checking flow at the patient interface, physically inspecting all connections, observing safe handling and stability of the unit, and assuring that flow rate is appropriate. The quantity of LOX in the portable should also be checked by observation of an indicator, such as a weight scale marker, etc..

An RC policy should outline the previous information and provide step-by-step instructions for LOX use. A checklist for maintenance and quality assurance is a definite plus.

12. The scenario presents the problem of poor mask fitting.

13. Corrective actions may include providing a protective dressing over the area of skin breakdown, treating the wound as indicated, and minimizing future problems of this nature by carefully resizing the mask or changing to a full face mask, nasal prong device, or other available product.

14.

Indications	Objectives	Interventions	Outcome Evaluations
Low oxygen indices	Assure oxygenation	Oxygen therapy	ABG/pulse oximetry/vital signs
Respiratory insufficiency/unstable ventilatory drive	Assure ventilation	NIPPV	ABG/pulse oximetry/vital signs/level of dyspnea
COPD	Improve exercise tolerance/promote self-care/improve breathing pattern, efficiency/promote pulmonary hygiene	Initiate pulmonary rehabilitation	Activity tolerance/breathing pattern/exercise testing/follow-up questionnaire
Wound (facial: associated with mask fit)	Promote wound healing indicated medications, treatments/ appropriately size mask/change application device as needed.	protective dressing/	No further skin lesions

15. An example of proper documentation of this problem should include the date and time of first observation of the problem, the patient's condition, corrective action, and subsequent plans. This documentation should occur via the patient's medical record, as well as in an incident report. The problem should also be reported to the United States Pharmacopeial Convention via the standard medical device problem reporting form.

16. Mr. Babson should meet the RC objectives of the RC plan. Other essential discharge assessments include general condition, cognitive level, economic factors, environmental factors, educational needs, and potential for reaching long-term goals.

17. Hazards of exercise testing include:[5]

    Electrocardiac abnormalities, severe desaturation, angina, hypotensive responses, lightheadedness, subjective complaints, hypertensive responses, mental confusion, headache, cyanosis, nausea, vomiting, muscle cramping, and hazards associated with equipment used, particularly electrical hazards.

18. The discharge plan should be expanded to include specific prescriptions for home care as well as cleaning and maintenance schedules. Precise dates should be included and the final "plan" documented.

19. A home oxygen prescription should include the device to be used, the liter flow, and duration or volume to be used. FiO_2 is included if applicable to the situation. The physician's signature should accompany the prescription. Follow-up should also be planned and assessments recorded.

20. Essential family factors of importance include adjustments and coping, education, practice, and evaluations of skills. A supportive healthcare environment should be maintained at all times.

21. Mr. Babson's educational plan:

    Points of emphasis:
    Equipment preparation and maintenance
    Prescription guidelines
    Hazards and complications
    Emergency plans
    Troubleshooting practice
    Monitoring progress and documentation
    Access to information/assistance
    Daily routines/ exercise

22. The RCP may make recommendations in the planning process, design the therapeutic plan, suggest home care providers, and perform follow-up assessments.

23. Assessments of financial capabilities, environmental conditions, family support/knowledge, and home care provider potential are needed. Community services could also be assessed.

24. Oxygen conserving devices:[6]

    Pulse dose method of delivery: delivering oxygen during inspiration only
    Reservoir cannula devices: provides a reservoir for minimizing oxygen waste
    Transtracheal oxygen therapy: direct administration of oxygen into the trachea via a thin catheter.

25. The initial home care visit should include an evaluation of the client's understanding of the plan and his ability to comply. The environment should also be assessed. All aspects of the educational plan (see question #21) should be assessed.

26. The physical assessments routinely performed are oximetry, auscultation, vital sign recording, observation, subjective data, level of dyspnea, (breathing pattern and accessory muscle use), color, dependent edema existence, and neck vein appearance.

27. The home environment should be assessed for:[7]

    Accessibility, equipment adaptability, and general condition (heating, electricity, space...)

28. The oxygen system will be assembled and checked as follows:
    For oxygen concentrators, the unit should be connected to the appropriate power outlet. Back-up

cylinders should be available. The unit is turned "on." Flowrate should be checked at the patient inter-face. Filters should be appropriately placed. The delivery device should be securely attached. FiO_2 should be checked as indicated. Regular and prescribed maintenance should be performed and docu-mented. Hours of usage should be observed and documented.

29. Mr. Babson should receive recommendations on safety issues, plan compliance, and availability of assistance. The plan should be reviewed at this point.

30. Mr. Babson should demonstrate all procedures as well as his understanding of all necessary informa-tion. Physical demonstration as well as written explanations are useful.

31. Mr. Babson should be visited weekly initially, then monthly to tri-monthly, or as otherwise indicated by need.

32. Home care follow-up should include documentation of the patient's physical and cognitive condition. Assessment compliance with the plan and equipment maintenance should occur. Environmental con-ditions should also be evaluated.

33. Backup supplies would include a manual resuscitator; extra ventilator circuits, adaptors, and parts; daily flow sheets; external battery; oxygen cylinders; emergency phone numbers; and humidity source if needed.

34. The home care RCP is a specialist in assessment and evaluation of the home care patient and environ-ment. The interventions are performed by the patient himself.

35 and 36.[8]

TRAVEL ARRANGEMENTS

When a patient contacts the office in need of oxygen and related equipment for travel purposes, obtain the following information from the patient:

1. Patient's home address and telephone number, including area code.
2. Destination address (as complete as possible)
3. Length of stay at destination (dates of arrival and departure)
4. Type of equipment needed.
5. Mode of travel.
6. Planned stops along the way, and length of stay at each stop.

Once this information has been obtained:

1. Locate area code of city of destination
2. Phone 1 (area code) 555-1212
3. Ask for phone number of any hospital in that town
4. Phone that hospital and ask for Respiratory Therapy Department or discharge planner
5. Inform Respiratory Therapist or discharge planner that a patient is coming to that area and would like a referral to an independent home care company.
6. Phone home care company and relay information on patient (date of arrival, place; etc.)
7. Question if they will:
   a. Prorate their charges
   b. Bill your company

If patient uses a cylinder, ask:
    a. Do they transfill
       1) steel portable
       2) aluminum portable

3) M-60 with American/Canadian standard safety system

If patient uses a liquid system, ask if they:
   a. Supply same type of system as patient has
   b. Provide portable

   8. Obtain complete name, address, phone, and contact person of company
   9. Inform patient of completed details
      a. Company name
      b. Contact person's name
      c. Company's complete address and phone number, including area code
      d. Your phone number, including area code

References

   1. Leger, P: Noninvasive positive pressure ventilation at home. Respiratory Care 39(5): 564, 1994.
   2. O' Ryan, J: Discharge planning for the respiratory patient. In: Lucas, J, et al: Home Respiratory Care. Appleton and Lange, Norwalk CT, 1988, p 235.
   3. Lucas, J, et al, p 75.
   4. Sleeper, G: Home oxygen therapy equipment. In: Lucas, J, et al, p 30.
   5. AARC clinical practice guideline: Exercise testing for evaluation of hypoxemia and/or desaturation. Respiratory Care 37(8): 908, 1992.
   6. Lucas, J, et al, p 82.
   7. Wyka, K and Scanlan, C: Respiratory home care. In: Scanlan, C: Fundamentals of Respiratory Care, ed 5, Mosby, 1995, p 1103.
   8. Sleeper, G: Traveling with Oxygen. In: Lucas, J, et al, p 106.

EXPERT OPINIONS FOR CHAPTER 16

1. RCPs trained in ACLS are likely to assume any role in ACLS. These are:[1]

   Primary Responsibilities
   Airway
   Ventilation
   Blood gases
   Instillation of endotracheal drugs

   Secondary Responsibilities
   Peripheral-vein catheter insertion
   Vascular drug infusion
   Defribillation (may become a primary responsibility with increased use of automated defribillators)

   Unlikely Responsibilities
   Central-line insertion
   Intraosseous needle insertion
   Intracardiax injection

2. Immediate needs are airway management, provision of ventilation, and circulation (ABCs).

3. The rhythm represents ventricular tachycardia. Because there is no palpable pulse present, this represents the need for rapid defibrillation as a priority. Therefore ACLS is indeed indicated.

4. The algorithm is as follows (see next page):[2]

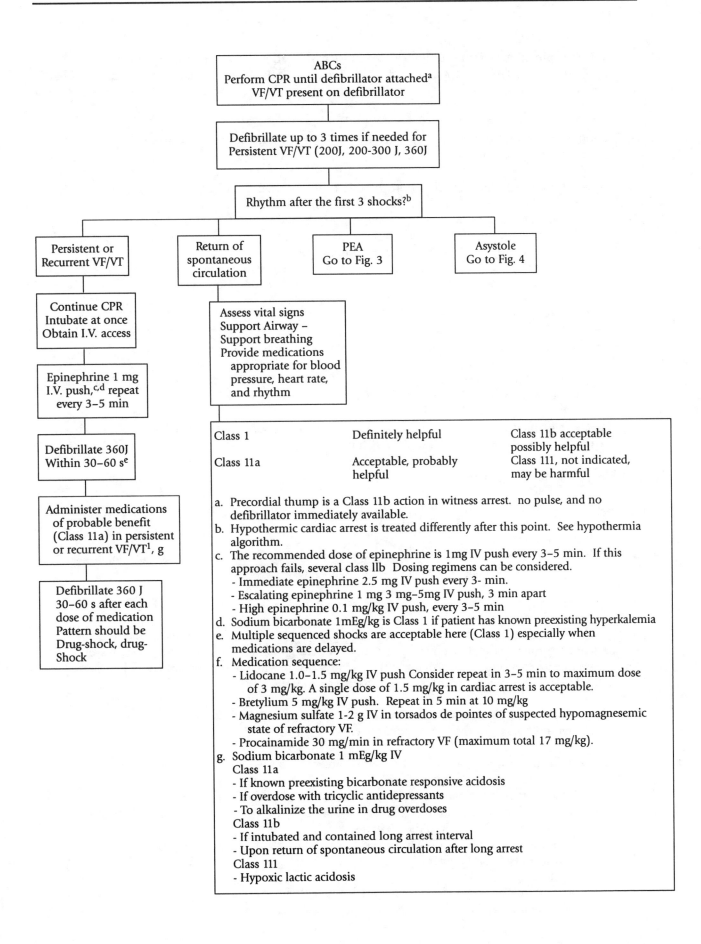

ABCs
Perform CPR until defibrillator attached[a]
VF/VT present on defibrillator

Defibrillate up to 3 times if needed for
Persistent VF/VT (200J, 200-300 J, 360J

Rhythm after the first 3 shocks?[b]

Persistent or
Recurrent VF/VT

Return of
spontaneous
circulation

PEA
Go to Fig. 3

Asystole
Go to Fig. 4

Continue CPR
Intubate at once
Obtain I.V. access

Epinephrine 1 mg
I.V. push,[c,d] repeat
every 3–5 min

Defibrillate 360J
Within 30–60 s[e]

Administer medications
of probable benefit
(Class 11a) in persistent
or recurrent VF/VT[1], g

Defibrillate 360 J
30–60 s after each
dose of medication
Pattern should be
Drug-shock, drug-
Shock

Assess vital signs
Support Airway –
Support breathing
Provide medications
   appropriate for blood
   pressure, heart rate,
   and rhythm

| Class 1 | Definitely helpful | Class 11b acceptable possibly helpful |
| Class 11a | Acceptable, probably helpful | Class 111, not indicated, may be harmful |

a. Precordial thump is a Class 11b action in witness arrest. no pulse, and no
   defibrillator immediately available.
b. Hypothermic cardiac arrest is treated differently after this point. See hypothermia
   algorithm.
c. The recommended dose of epinephrine is 1mg IV push every 3–5 min. If this
   approach fails, several class llb Dosing regimens can be considered.
   - Immediate epinephrine 2.5 mg IV push every 3- min.
   - Escalating epinephrine 1 mg 3 mg–5mg IV push, 3 min apart
   - High epinephrine 0.1 mg/kg IV push, every 3–5 min
d. Sodium bicarbonate 1mEg/kg is Class 1 if patient has known preexisting hyperkalemia
e. Multiple sequenced shocks are acceptable here (Class 1) especially when
   medications are delayed.
f. Medication sequence:
   - Lidocane 1.0–1.5 mg/kg IV push Consider repeat in 3–5 min to maximum dose
     of 3 mg/kg. A single dose of 1.5 mg/kg in cardiac arrest is acceptable.
   - Bretylium 5 mg/kg IV push. Repeat in 5 min at 10 mg/kg
   - Magnesium sulfate 1-2 g IV in torsados de pointes of suspected hypomagnesemic
     state of refractory VF.
   - Procainamide 30 mg/min in refractory VF (maximum total 17 mg/kg).
g. Sodium bicarbonate 1 mEg/kg IV
   Class 11a
   - If known preexisting bicarbonate responsive acidosis
   - If overdose with tricyclic antidepressants
   - To alkalinize the urine in drug overdoses
   Class 11b
   - If intubated and contained long arrest interval
   - Upon return of spontaneous circulation after long arrest
   Class 111
   - Hypoxic lactic acidosis

5. Neck and spinal injuries must be anticipated in such a situation. The airway should be opened using the jaw thrust maneuver as opposed to the head tilt-chin lift. Head and neck immobility are essential, as is careful body movement in general. The intention should be not to extend any possible neck or head injury.

6. Endotracheal administration, intraosseous delivery, and intracardiac access are acceptable routes for several of the drugs. The following apply to endotracheal administration:[3]

   - Endrotracheal drug administration should not be considered a first-line therapy during cardiac arrest; this route should only be used if venous access cannot be secured.
   - At least for epinephrine, an appropriate endotracheal dose is 10 times the intravenous dose.
   - No clear superiority has been shown for instillation through a catheter, and, therefore, direct instillation into the endotracheal tube should be used.
   - The dose should be diluted to 10 mL with either normal saline or water.
   - Five rapid insufflations should be used after endotracheal drug.

7. Yes, see question 6.

8. At this point, tracheostomy or cricoidotomy appear to be the likely options.

9. Potential complications associated with removal of an esophageal obturator include vomiting with or without aspiration and potential loss of airway patency in general.

10. The assessments indicate that a left-sided, traumatic pneumothorax has occurred. Flail chest is likely. A chest tube should be inserted into the left chest.

11. The Glasgow coma rating is 3.

12. Other scoring systems include the APACHE (acute physiology and chronic health evaluation) and SAPS (simplified acute physiology score).

13. Verification procedures include auscultation for the presence of bilateral breath sounds, capnography checks, visual inspection, and general observation of the patient.

14. Tracheostomy is indicated by the inability to intubate orally due to the presence of laryngeal edema.

15. Based on the history of massive chest trauma, hemoptysis, and assymetrical chest movement, the patient has probably developed a pneumothorax or hemopneumothorax. With positive pressure ventilation, the affected side is (or perhaps both sides are) filling with air and possibly blood. Because little air and blood are leaving, the thorax is approaching its elastic limit.

16. Any one or more of the following may have resulted from the trauma and caused a pneumothorax or hemopneumothorax. This list is not exhaustive.

    - A bronchus was torn, allowing air to enter directly into the pleural space (bronchopleural fistula) instead of going into the parenchyma.
    - Alveoli were ruptured, allowing air to enter into the pleural space.
    - A broken rib punctured both pleural layers and provided a passageway from the lung parenchyma or even bronchi directly into the pleural space.
    - A laceration completely through the thoracic wall (caused by the automobile or a broken rib), allowing outside air to enter the pleural space. Tissue acting as a "flap valve" would prevent air from leaving.
    - Torn, cut, or punctured blood vessels are likely with all of the above producing a hemopneumothorax

- A torn, cut, or punctured major blood vessel (pulmonary artery or vein, vena cava, aorta) with or without any of the above could produce a hemothorax sufficient to increase the difficulty of ventilating the patient.

17. The ECG represents sinus bradycardia with a heart rate of 56–58 BPM. Atropine should be administered IV.

18. Sinus rhythm with HR = 65–75 BPM is noted. No new treatment should begin.

19. An example ventilator flow sheet:[5]

Objectives	Interventions/Settings	Expected Outcomes
Assure oxygenation	Supplemental O_2 via vent. (FiO_2 = 1.00)	PaO_2 > 55 mmHg.
Assure ventilation	PPV with:	$PaCO_2$ = 20 mmHg.
	RR = >16 (to intentionally hyperventilate) Vt = 750 mL	
Maintain patent airway	Provide suctioning and tracheostomy care	Patient/airway/no infection

20. The patient ventilator system should be checked "on a scheduled basis (institution-specific) as well as prior to obtaining ABG, prior to obtaining hemodynamic or PFT data, following any change in ventilator settings, as soon as possible following an acute deterioration of the patient's condition, and any time that ventilator performance is questionable."[4]

21. In addition to verifying all ventilator settings and assuring appropriate mechanical operation of all equipment (humidifier, oxygen analyzer, temperature regulation, etc.) as recommended by the AARC Clinical Practice Guideline,[4] specific serial assessment of this patient should include the following items. It is vital to include in the assessment process all changes in patient parameters that have occurred since the previous check.

   - General patient appearance
   - Breath sounds
   - Chest movement
   - Airway secretions
   - Tracheostomy tube cuff pressure, tube position and stability
   - Patient respiratory movement and synchrony with the ventilator
   - Inhaled and exhaled tidal volumes (is there air leaking through the chest tube? How much? Has it changed?)
   - Static compliance
   - Airway resistance
   - Oxygenation status (continuous oximetry, arterial blood gases [ABGs] as indicated)
   - Ventilatory status (continuous end-tidal capnography, ABGs as indicated)

22. Ventilator circuits using nebulizers as humidifiers require 24 hr changing. Circuits employing heated humidifiers (cascade, HME, or wicks) may be changed at an interval of >5 days. HMEs should be changed every 24 hr. Circuits should be changed to maintain a clean appearance.[6]

23. Airway care of this patient would entail regular suctioning, cleaning of the exterior (and interior cannula if used) and stomal areas with a hydrogen peroxide and water mixture, and changing or cleaning the securing device (e.g, changing the trach-tube tape). Any bronchial drainage procedures needed to maintain airway patency should occur as indicated. All procedures should be documented appropriately as well.

24. FFB assembly and operational verification checklist:

   __Patient parameters assessed
   __Bronchoscope channel assessed, leak test passed

__Equipment is clean and has had recommended disinfection/sterilization
__All attachable devices operate smoothly and correctly
__All monitors are functional and accessible
__All infection control guidelines are followed
__All necessary equipment, medication, and supplies are present (supply checklist should accompany)

25. The serious complications that Elle Carey is at risk for are:[7]

Adverse effects of medication used during the procedure
Hypoxemia, hypercarbia
Wheezing
Hypotension
Laryngospasm, bradycardia, or other vagal phenomenon
Mechanical complications (epistaxis, pneumothorax, and hemoptysis)
Increased airway resistance
Death
Infection for healthcare workers, the patient, and other patients
Cross-contamination of specimens

26. Supplies needed for insertion of a pulmonary artery catheter include:

The catheter (multilumen/fluid filled)
Heparinized saline fluid source/ pressurized
A transducer
A monitor
Dressing materials/ securing devices (?sutures)

27. Operational verification of a pulmonary artery catheter system would include flushing the line for patency, damping, and leaking and checking all connections, calibration procedures, and checklists for documenting equipment, continuous flow, time/date, and location of the line.

28. For the safe transport of this patient the RCP must gather all necessary supplies, monitor the patient, maintain the integrity of the patient/ventilator system, and prevent any known hazards from occurring.

29. RC plan:

Objectives	Interventions (Include Monitors)	Expected Outcomes
1. Assure airway patency, ABG ventilation and oxygenation	PPV via tracheal tube	Maintenance of adequate and clear CXR
2. Promote resolution of pneumothorax and re-expansion of lungs	Chest drainage system maintenance	Resolution of pneumothorax/ clear CXR
3. Monitor and maintain normal hemodynamic values	Maintenance of PA catheter system	Hemodynamics within norm ranges, no evidence of pulmonary edema
4. Promote neurologic recovery	Monitor ICP and neurologic exam, prevent increase in ICP	ICP < no evidence of extension of injuries.
5. Prevent infection and promote patient safety	Use aseptic techniques/follow infection control guidelines	Patient is free of infection/ injury

30. The following items will need to be removed, disinfected (or disguarded), and then replaced: resuscitation bag, oxygen tubing, masks, airways, IV supplies, suction requipment, ECG lead attachments, and linens.

31. The hemodynamic data indicate that left ventricular failure is occurring.

32. A combination of intraoperative stressors, combined with an increase in fluids during surgery, and the head injury with its potential to manifest pulmonary edema, all contribute to this problem.

33. Furosemide is indicated for diuresis at this time.

34. The end of the chest tube should be submerged in sterile water and/or then attached to a new chest drainage unit.

35. Effects of maintaining a chest drainage system should be monitored by the patient's vital signs, physical appearance, ECG, and auscultation. Further evaluation should be an ongoing process.

36. In an instance such as this the practitioner should be as tactful and kind as possible. This question should be referred to the physician since the nature of the information requires a comprehensive and prognostic scope. All means to assure the father that his daughter is receiving excellent care and is being treated kindly as well as carefully should be employed.

37. With high cervical injuries the victim is likely to experience partial function of the shoulder and elbow with paralysis elsewhere.[8]

38. Maintenance of ICP occurs via:[9]
    - elevation of the head of the bed (15–30°)
    - avoidance of hip, waist, and neck flexion
    - avoidance of head rotation
    - minimization of activities
    - performance of suctioning only as needed

39. If the PA catheter tip was positioned higher than the monitoring transducer, the monitor would read erroneously higher than the actual measurement.

40. Yes, since intentional hyperventilation is effective for approximately 8 hours only, and this time has elapsed.[10]

41. At this point the patient is stable with all cardiopulmonary data shown to be in the normal range. Signs of neurologic recovery are also noted by the pupil reactivity and ability to focus.

42. Conditions for successful transition may be classified into three categories: physiologic stability, clinical stability, and social/psychological stability.

Conditions of physiologic stability
- Other organ systems are stable
- There is an absence of acute infections
- An optimal acid-base and metabolic status can be maintained
- Ventilator parameters: FiO_2 stable and 40%; PEEP, 10 cm H_2O; the time on and off the ventilator is stable

Conditions of clinical stability
- There is an absence of significant sustained dyspnea or severe dyspneic episodes or tachypnea
- Patient maintains acceptable arterial blood gas levels with FiO_2, 40%
- There is an absence of life-threatening cardiac dysfunction or arrhythmias
- There is an ability to clear secretions
- There is evidence of gag/cough reflex or a protected airway
- There is an absence of significant aspiration
- Patient has a tracheostomy (as opposed to a nasal tracheal tube)

Conditions of social/psychological stability
- The patient must desire to be at home
- The patient's family must desire to have the patient at home
- The patient and family must have the ability to learn and perform necessary care.
- The psychological health of the patient must be stable.
- The psychological health of the primary caregivers must be stable and any other members of the household must be accepting and supportive.
- There must be social support mechanisms in place outside the household.
- There must be adequate financial support.
- There must be an adequate physical environment.
- There must be health professional support.
- There must be technical support.
- There must be community support.

43. Essential components of the long-term MV plan include all of the aspects noted in question 42 with a checklist breakdown of daily and weekly tasks, including who is responsible for each.

44. Without the acceptance and support of all members of the household, the patient is placed at great risk in a home environment. In this case, an optimal setting might be a long-term care facility or a home-like environment with professional caregivers.

    Oral (or nasal) endotracheal intubation is not compatible with home care. In addition to problems associated with stabilizing the tube, reintubation in the event of extubation or tube damage is not available, and tissue damage due to the presence of the tube in upper airway and the stabilizing mechanism (tape or straps) may be severe.

    If the patient did not regain consciousness:

    She could not participate in the decision to be at home.
    She would require additional, continuous monitoring (heart, respiration, oxygenation, and ventilation)
    She would require continuous observation

    None of these are likely to promote a positive outcome for the patient in the long term.

References

1. Hess, D Ravikumar A: Methods of emergency drug administration. Respiratory Care 40(5): 503, 1995.
2. American Heart Association. Guidelines for cardiopulmonary resuscitation and emergency cardiac care. JAMA 268:2213, 1992.
3. Hess, et al. p. 510.
4. AARC clinical practice guideline: Patient-ventilator system checks. Respiratory Care 37(8): 884, 1992.
5. Kacmarek, R: Management of the patient-mechanical ventilator system. In Kacmarek, R and Pierson D: Foundations of Respiratory Care. Churchill-Livingston, 1992, pp. 989-990.
6. AARC clinical practice guideline: Ventilator circuit changes. Respiratory Care 39(8):800, 1994.
7. AARC clinical practice guidelines: Fiberoptic bronchoscopy assisting. Respiratory Care 38: 1173.
8. Smeltzer, C and Bare, B: Brunner and Suddarth's Textbook of Medical-Surgical Nursing, ed 7. JB Lippincott, Philadelphia, 1992, p 1739.
9. Schenk, E: Management of persons with common neurologic manifestations. In Phipps, et al: Medical Surgical Nursing. Mosby, 1991, p 1800.
10. Severinghaus, J: Role of cerebrospinal fluid pH in normalization of cerebral blood flow in chronic hpocapnia. Acta Neurol, Scand 14:116-120, 1965.

EXPERT OPINIONS FOR CHAPTER 17

1. and 2. The factors that place the fetus at risk for physical problems are:
   fetal factors—postmaturity, late fetal heart decelerations, fetal scalp pH of 7.26.
   maternal factors—primagravida, dystocia, presence of meconium in amniotic fluid, vaginal bleeding, elevated blood pressure, peripheral edema, hyper-reflexia, proteinurea.

3. Preeclampsia is indicated by the data.

4. Fetal asphyxia is likely, as evidenced by the late heart decelerations and the pH of 7.26.

5. The late decelerations indicate fetal distress.

6. The RCP should assemble and make ready all supplies, equipment, and resources required for a high-risk delivery.

7. The action plan in this case would consist of the overview of resuscitation in the delivery room (see Figure 17-2) combined with careful monitoring of the mother.

8. The infant's oro/naso pharynx should be suctioned before the body is delivered. This may prevent aspiration of the meconium during the first breath.

9. Magnesium sulfate is an anticonvulsive medication and is used to prevent seizures.

10. Suction equipment should be assembled according to manufacturer's guidelines, assuring that all equipment (vacuum source, regulator, container, connecting tubing, and catheter(s)) are gathered. The regulator should be observed for proper function by a test aspiration, and all connections should be checked. Equipment should be handled aseptically.

11. See question 12.

12. Suctioning the meconium prior to delivery of the body may prevent aspiration during the first breath. After delivery the trachea should be intubated with the largest endotracheal tube possible. Suction may be applied directly to the endotracheal tube. The ET tube should be withdrawn and examined for meconium. This process may need to be repeated until there is no or very little meconium seen. Careful and thorough oxygenation should occur via 100% oxygen blown by the patient's face during the procedure. PPV may then be initiated and subsequent resuscitative and therapeutic actions.[1]

13. Resuscitation supplies:[2]

   Emergency medications
   Face masks
   Oxygen supplies
   Suction supplies
   Resuscitation bags
   Laryngoscopes and extra bulbs, scissors, gloves
   Stylet
   Endotracheal and tracheostomy tubes
   Oral airways
   Intravascular access supplies
   Defibrillator
   Radiant warmer

> Stethoscope
> Tape, alcohol wipes, stopcocks, syringes, needles
> Umbilical artery catheterization supplies
> Feeding tubes
> Monitors

14. Daily quality assurance procedures should be enacted to assure that all emergency supplies are ready at all times. Checklists for content of supply carts and performance evaluations of healthcare workers' skills are essential. These check-offs should be performed on a scheduled basis according to institutional policy. The schedule and duties should be clearly understood by all.

15. Warming, drying, and stimulating the infant may be all that is needed in some instances. Therefore it is essential to initiate resuscitation with these steps. They are the first steps of the sequenced process.

16. APGAR scoring of 3 could occur as: heart rate of 60 with no respiratory efforts, grimacing, some muscle flexion, and a pale blue body color.

17. Either self-inflating or non-self-inflating resuscitation bags are used. In-line pressure manometers are used to monitor the peak airway pressures generated during ventilations.

18. The neonate receiving resuscitation efforts is evaluated as to respiratory rate, heart rate, color, muscle tone, and reflex abilities.

19. Endotracheal intubation is preferred in the case of meconium aspiration, because bag mask ventilation may force meconium deeper into the trachea. The endotracheal tube is suctioned before ventilations are initiated.

20. Neonatal anatomical features that predispose to difficult intubation are the infant's relatively larger head, proportionally smaller nares, large and highly vascular adenoid tissue, and relatively larger tongue and rounder jaw. The infant larynx lie higher in the neck and are more funnel shaped than adults. The infant epiglottis is longer and more horizontal. The infant mucosa is thin and easily traumatized. Stimulation of the infant larynx may result in prolonged apnea.[3]

21. The procedure for neonatal oral intubation:[4]

> Position the patient (supine, sniffing position if possible)
> Apply 100% oxygen (2–5 minutes)
> Ventilate via resuscitation bag and mask if needed
> Initiate sedation, anesthetic, neuromuscular blockers, as indicated
> Cricoid pressure may be applied
> Open mouth (use forefinger and thumb in a scissor motion)
> Insert laryngoscope
> Select ET tube
> Place ET tube in right hand
> Insert via right side of mouth
> Advance until tip is correctly positioned (2 cm above the carina)
> Attempts at intubation should be limited to 30 seconds
> Secure tube in place
> Assure ventilation/assure oxygenation
> Assess and monitor patient

22. A size 4.0 mm oral endotracheal tube would be a likely first choice for this case.

23. Endotracheal tube placement may be assessed by capnometry, auscultation, chest radiograph, and physical observation.

24. The RCP transporting Mort Merten will need assistance from other RCPs or health providers to assemble and check all the needed equipment for this child. The RCP will also need to perform a thorough physical assessment. A respiratory care plan will also need to be devised.

25. The RCP would need to ask others to help and delegate necessary tasks to them.

26. A left-sided pneumothorax is detected.

27. Asymmetrical chest movement, lack of left-sided breath sounds, the presence of respiratory distress, and the patient's history all combine to support the potential for pneumothorax.

28. Additional assessments that are needed for confirmation of the pneumothorax are a chest radiograph and continued general assessments, possibly including arterial blood gases.

29. Chest tube insertion is indicated.

30. Short inspiratory times allow for longer exhalation times. Thus, prevention of further air trapping due to the obstructive nature of meconium in the airways is promoted.

31. The ABG indicates respiratory acidosis with hypoxemia.

32. Recommended PPV settings:

    Peak airway pressure = 40 cmH$_2$0
    PEEP = 5 cm H$_2$0
    FiO$_2$ = 1.00
    RR = 60 BPM
    I:E ratio = 1:1.5
    Inspiratory time = .4 sec.

    Consider high frequency ventilation if persistent air leak occurs.

33. Increasing PEEP levels without corresponding changes in peak airway pressures would decrease alveolar ventilation (by a tidal volume reduction) and thus would produce increases in PaCO$_2$ levels.

34. Transillumination is the process of using a high intensity light probe, placed on the infant's chest, to observe the lucent area shining around the probe tip. The lucent area should be evenly spread in approximately a 2–3 cm circular pattern. Intrathoracic air is detected when the size of the lucent area increases and may change pattern from circular to irregular.[5]

35. To check the TCM one should allow appropriate warm up time, perform calibration (2 points), observe proper handling of probes, and note the temperature of the probe. Then as always, one should observe the performance of the instrument for stable readings that are realistic.

36. Quality assurance for TCMs consists of regularly scheduled calibration checks analysis of control substances, regular maintenance, documentation of performance of the instrument, and recordkeeping of all QA data.

37. TCM probe sites should be changed every 2–4 hours.[6]

38. TCM probe sites should be changed if burns or blistering are noted.

39. Desirable TCM probe site locations are flat, nonbony areas of the body.

40.

Objectives	Interventions	Indications/Rationales	Evaluations
1. Assure ventilation	PPV	Respiratory failure	ABG, physical inspection, auscultation, WOB, oxygen and ventilation indices
2. Assure oxygenation	Supplemental oxygen	Hypoxemia	ABG, oximetry oxygen indices
3. Maintain airway patency	Artificial airway	Potential for airway obstruction	Observation, capnometry, auscultation, oxygenation/ and ventilation indices
4. Prevent infection	Observation of good infection control techniques	At risk for infection	Vital signs, WBC, physical observation
5. Promote patient safety	Compliance with standard safety practices	Potential for injury	Observe for no injuries

41. A: collection chamber, B: water seal chamber, C: suction control chamber.

42. Mort Merten exhibits good response to chest tube insertion as evidenced by improved oxygenation and ventilation, no signs of respiratory distress, improved chest expansion, breath sounds, color improvement, and stability of vital signs.

43. It appears there is a patent ductus arteriosus.

44. If conditions worsen, possible strategies would include high frequency ventilation, extracorporeal membrane oxygenation, or nitric oxide ventilation.

45.

	Risks	Benefits
ECMO	Seizures, intraventricular hemorrhage, pulmonary hemorrhage, pneumothorax, infection, dialysis, hemolysis, hypertension, abnormal creatinine values, electrolyte imbalance, hyperbilirubinemia, cardiac problems, bleeding from insertion sites, and mechanical/technical problems	Improved oxygenation, improved ventilation, improved survival when conventional means fail.
High Frequency Ventilation	Air trapping, mechanical/technical problems, tracheitis, hypotension, intraventricular hemorrhage, and cardiac dysfunction	Same as above
PPV with nitric-oxide	Acute respiratory distress, impaired development, IVH, all complications associated with PPV	Decreased pulmonary resistance, decreased R-L shunting, increased pulmonary blood flow (leading to improved oxygenation/ventilation/ survival)

46. The RCP can promote parental coping by exhibiting caring, comforting, and supportive gestures toward the parent. Promotion of the parenting role by including the father in some levels of care and communication will also benefit. The RCP may promote his or her own coping by under-standing that this is not unusual behavior for a parent under this stress. The RCP should not personalize the father's anger. It is also wise to perform self-checks, assessing one's own stress level and practicing stress management/relief.[7]

47. The plan may be adjusted as follows:

Objectives	Interventions	Indications/Rationales	Evaluations
1. Assure ventilation	Monitor	Spontaneous breathing	Observe ABG as needed
2. Assure oxygenation	Monitor	Stable oxygenation status	Oximetry PRN.
3. Maintain airway	Monitor	Patency maintained by patient	Observe patency
4. Prevent infection	Observation of good infection control techniques	At risk for infection	Vital signs, WBC, physical observation
5. Promote patient safety	Compliance with standard safety practices	Potential for injury	Observe for no injuries
6. Resolve pulmonary infiltrates	Chest physical therapy	RUL infiltrate	CXR, physical examination, lab values

48. The AARC clinical practice guidelines that may be observed for use in such a case as this are:

- Postural drainage therapy
- Oxygen therapy
- Pulse oximetry
- Patient ventilator system checks
- Humidification during mechanical ventilation
- Selection of aerosol delivery device
- Arterial blood gas sampling
- Use of positive airway pressure adjuncts to bronchial hygiene therapy
- Endotracheal suctioning of mechanically ventilated adults and children with artificial airways
- Transport of the mechanically ventilated patient
- Fiberoptic bronchoscopy assisting
- Resuscitation in acute care hospitals
- Ventilator circuit changes
- Neonatal time-triggered pressure-limited time-cycled mechanical ventilation
- Application of continuous positive airway pressure to neonates via nasal prongs or nasophyaryngeal tube
- Capillary blood gas sampling neonatal and pediatric patients
- Transcutaneous blood gas monitoring for neonatal and pediatric patients
- Infant/toddler pulmonary function tests
- Management of airway emergencies
- Capnography/capnometry during mechanical ventilation
- Discharge planning for the respiratory care patient

References

1. Whittaker, K: Comprehensive Perinatal and Pediatric Respiratory Care. Delmar NY, 1992. pp 372–373.
2. Whittaker, p 90.
3. Smith-Wenning, K. et al: Neonatal and pediatric respiratory care. In Scanlan, C: Egan's Fundamentals of Respiratory Care. Mosby, St. Louis, 1995, p 998.
4. Barnhart, S and Czervinske, M: Clinical Handbook of Perinatal and Pediatric Respiratory Care. WB Saunders, Philadelphia, 1995, p 383.
5. Barnhart, et al, p 226.
6. Barnhart, et al, p 325.
7. Barnhart, et al, p 6.

EXPERT OPINIONS FOR CHAPTER 18

1. The factors presenting that indicate decelerated lung maturity in twin B include prematurity (29 wk gestations), very low birth weight (1020 g), maternal age (15 yr), and mild maternal diabetes.

2. As mentioned, the maternal risks are young maternal age and the presence of diabetes.

3. Terbutaline was used as a tocolytic agent in this case to slow or stop the mother's premature uterine contractions. Other such medications include ritodrine, magnesium sulfate, and nifedipine.

4. Type II fetal heart decelerations (heart rate < 120 min), occur after uterine contractions begin and return to baseline sometime after the contraction ends. This type of deceleration is commonly secondary to uteroplacental insufficiency and may lead to fetal asphyxia. Asphyxia may also be reflected by fetal scalp pH of less then 7.24.[1] With the evidence presented, asphyxia may not be ruled out in this case. Quick and decisive action is required.

5. RDS is defined by the premature condition, the clinical presentation of respiratory distress at birth and the L/S ratio of less than 2:1 accompanied by the low birth weight. Further evidence would include a CXR revealing granularities often called ground glass. Air bronchograms may also be noted.

6. This infant has an APGAR score of 1.

    Scoring:
    1 for HR present
    0 for apnea
    0 for central cyanosis
    0 for flaccid extremities
    0 for lack of response to stimuli

7. The initial steps in neonatal resuscitation are:[2]

    1. Dry and warm the infant after placing in a radiant warmer
    2. Place the infant in the supine position, suction nares and mouth with bulb syringe
    3. Tactile stimulation of the heels or back if apnea persists
    4. Bag-valve-mask ventilation if apnea still persists

8. This child of 29 wk gestation and weighing 1020 g would require a 3.0-mm ID endotracheal tube. Assessments of the airway and chest should follow the intubation to assure adequacy of the airway. Commercially available surfactants that are common today are human surfactant, Surfactant-TA, Survanta, (both are bovine extractions), Curosurf (porcine) and Exosurf (synthetic). According to manufacturers' guidelines, surfactant is delivered endotracheally, with some modifications for particular brands, in the dose of 4–5 mL/kg. The infant is placed in various drainage positions to facilitate administration to all lobes. Positive pressure ventilation is maintained throughout administration.[3]

9. Surfactant is indicated in this case by the gestational age and low birth weight. The lecithin: sphingomyelin ratio of less than 2 also indicates surfactant deficiency. Another indicator is the absence of phosphotidylglycerol. This deficiency along with the initial assessments supports the diagnosis of RDS, and the RDS diagnosis itself is an indication for surfactant replacement.[3]

10. On the next page is a completed map about surfactant.

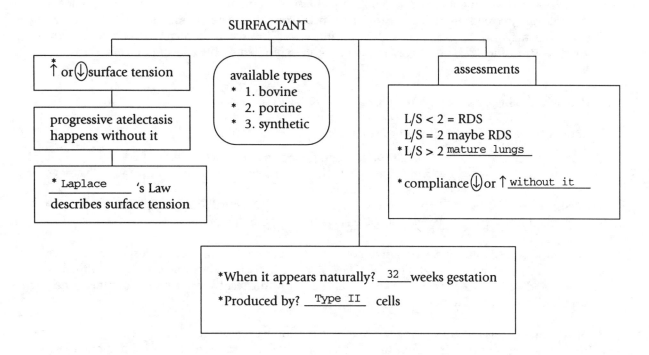

11. The indications for instituting NP- CPAP in this case are the occurrence of RDS in combination with spontaneous breathing.

12. Discussion should focus on the relationship and rationale linking the interventions to the outcomes. "If" and "then" statements may serve as a starting point, with development of ideas and sequencing of of events expanding the discussion. For example "if" oxygenation via supplement oxygen and CPAP will provide the environment for achieving adequate oxygenation (and already having adequate ventilation) "then" the effects of CPAP, namely increasing mean airway pressure, improving ventilation distribution, preventing alveolar collapse or early closure, reducing airway resistance, increasing static compliance, increasing FRC, and improving gas and fluid distribution in the lung, must combine to produce the outcome. This type of structured discussion allows attention to be focused on the interrelationship between a modality, its physiologic effects, and the outcome of treatment. This process could continue focusing on the other interventions: monitoring, stimulating when needed, providing/assessing pulmonary hygiene, providing airway care, and maintaining neutral thermal environment.

13. Assessments indicating achievement of the RC objectives include:

Arterial Blood Gas Data

- PaO_2 between 50 and 90 torr
- $PaCO_2$ between 35 and 45 torr
- pH between 7.35 and 7.45

Other Assessments

- Negative CXR
- Stable vital signs
- Clear breath sounds
- Stable hemodynamics
- Minimal secretion production
- No equipment malfunctions during use
- Maintenance of lowest mechanical ventilation parameters (e.g., respiratory frequency, airway pressures, positive expiratory pressures)

14. The optimal responses to interventions would include achievement of the expected outcomes: adequate oxygenation/ventilation during spontaneous breathing, clear breath sounds, negative CXR, stable vital signs, stable hemodynamics, minimal sputum production. (Note that body temperature is characteristically included in vital signs.)

15. Negative responses might include the inability to resume spontaneous breathing, thus dependence on technologic interventions. Other negative responses would be related to the interventions. Some negative events may include increased work of breathing, cardiovascular problems, equipment malfunctions, airway difficulties, infections, and gastric system problems. The list could increase significantly if specific instances were to be cited.

16. Heat loss can be prevented in the following ways:

Route of Heat Loss	Method of Prevention
- Conduction	- Warm all surfaces and materials in contact with the child
- Convection	- Warm the air circulating around or near the infant; use radiant warmers; use heated humidifiers
- Radiation	- Keep all surfaces warm that may indirectly contact the patient
- Evaporation	- Provide 100% relative humidity to the infant

17. Transcutaneous monitoring is performed on a continuous basis as opposed to a spot check schedule, in order to perform trend analysis on the data. Because transcutaneous values correlate with arterial values, and do not match them, it is important to follow the results over a period of time, rather than simply check them periodically.[4]

18. Airway care of this patient would include airway suctioning,[5] cleaning of the exterior portion of the tube, changing and cleaning of the tubing adaptor, visual inspection of the airway and oral cavity, cleaning of the skin area around the mouth and nose, oral hygiene procedures, changing of the tape or nasopharyngeal tube holder, and continuous assessment of the airway. Several bronchial hygiene methods may be combined with simple airway care to facilitate secretion mobilization. (This topic could be expanded to include discussion on airways, suctioning, bronchial hygiene, and assessment.)

19. The plan appears complete and appropriate. More specificity and detail regarding protocol and policy may be helpful.

20. Positive pressure ventilation is indicated on day 1 at 2:00PM by the noted increase in $PaCO_2$ with a downward trend in the pH. These ABG findings are accompanied by signs of respiratory distress, namely grunting, flaring, and retractions.

21. Time-triggered, pressure-limited, time-cycled ventilation (TPTV) is described as a type of ventilation wherein mandatory breaths are initiated by an elapsed time interval (time triggered), a preset pressure determines the level of pressure to be reached during each breath (pressure-limited), and inspiration ends when a specified time period has elapsed (time-cycled).[6] Some emphasis should be made regarding the fact that the tidal volume is variable in TPTV.

22. Ventilator settings are within normal limits for the infant.

23. On day 2 the stools are found to be guaiac positive, the abdomen is distended, and the WBC is in the high range. Oxygenation is remaining poor. Gas bubbles are seen by radiograph in the intestinal wall.

24. Collectively these data indicate that necrotizing enterocolitis (NEC) is present.

25. Increases in oxygen demand are likely to occur with NEC. This demand is associated with the increased metabolic activity involved in the infectious process. Increases in delivered oxygen may facilitate mucosal healing as well as general improvement.

26. On day 3 the cardiac murmur and $PtcO_2$ gradient indicate that the ductus arteriosus remains open (PDA).

27. Indomethicin was requested to close the PDA. Its use is not favored when an infection is present. (Remember that NEC is present)[7]

28. The weaning progression appears appropriate.

29. Objectives and outcomes for ventilator weaning plan.

Objectives	Expected Outcomes/Rationale
1. Maintain oxygenation/ventilation	- Oxygenation indicators (PaO_2, SaO_2, CaO_2, oximetry, heart rate) and ventilation indicators ($PaCO_2$, work of breathing, respiratory rate, pulmonary mechanics, appearance, breathing pattern) are appropriate for the patient.
2. Decrease levels of mechanical - ↓ respiratory frequency - ↓ cycling pressures - ↓ PEEP levels - ↓ FiO_2	- Infant maintains oxygenation/ventilation while spontaneously breathing room air
3. Discontinue artificial airway dependence and use	- Infant clears secretions - Breath sounds are clear - Chest radiograph is negative
4. Monitor continuously for positive and negative events	- Documentation is complete, accurate, and timely
5. Provide services needed to	- Infant receives increased levels of support as indicated by maintain safety assessments. Plan is regulated as needed. Circuit changes and system checks are performed as per policy references 8 and 9

30. Baby Hicks is likely to be diagnosed as having bronchopulmonary dysplasia (BPD) upon discharge. The CXR reveals cystic lesions, the ABGs show continuing hypoxemia without supplemental oxygen, and the infant's breath sounds reveal wheezing. All of these assessments indicate that BPD is present. Further evidence for the diagnosis is found in the patient history of exposure to oxygen, positive pressure, and occurrence of a PDA.[3] *Suggestion:* Have students create a "map" or chart of all of the assessments in this case, making note of values and norms. Encourage examination of other assessment "maps."

31. Home therapy indications are as follows:

Intervention	Indication
Oxygen via nasal cannula at .4l/min	- $PaO_2 < 55$ while breathing room air using an oxygen concentrator in the home and portable for back-up and ambulation
Aerosolized bronchodilator via small volume nebulizer (SVN) q6 hr.	- presence of wheezing
Ongoing pulmonary assessment	- infant at risk for developing pulmonary complications (e.g., infection, airway problems, atelectasis)

32. The oxygenation status of the infant could easily and safely be monitored via oximetry as well as physical assessment of vital signs, appearance, and activity tolerance. The ventilation status could be evaluated by monitoring respiratory rate and pattern, auscultation of the chest, physical examination, and a spot check capillary blood gas to monitor patient progress or evaluate a change in patient status.

33. The home RC plan:[10,11,12]

Intervention	Indication
- Oxygen via nasal cannula at .4l/min	- PaO_2 < 55 while breathing room air using an oxygen concentrator in the home (i.e., infection, airway obstruction, atelectasis) and portable compressed gas for back-up and ambulation
- Aerosolized bronchodilator via small volume nebulizer (SVN) q6 hr.	- Presence of wheezing
- Ongoing pulmonary assessment	- Infant at risk for developing pulmonary complications

- Monitor:
   oximetry
   capillary blood gases (strictly PRN)
   physical exam/general observation
   vital signs
   auscultation	

- Regulate plan	
- Education/instructions to parents	

Objectives

1. Maintain PaO_2 > 55torr (SpO_2 > 85%)
2. Diminish/prevent presence of wheezing
3. Prevent complications/ensure safety in the home
4. Provide parents with education about pathophysiology and equipment

Expected outcomes

- Baby Hicks is without dyspnea
- Cough is effective
- Breath sounds are clear
- Vital signs are stable
- Infant is as mobile as possible
- Parents demonstrate skill in equipment set-up and use, as well as knowledge relating to the child's condition, the equipment, the oxygen, and all potential complications.
- Equipment functions properly

References

1. Whitaker, K: Comprehensive Perinatal and Pediatric Respiratory Care. Delmar, NY, 1992, p 40.
2. Bloom, RS and Cropley, C: Textbook of Neonatal Resuscitation. Evanston, IL: American Heart Association/American Academy of Pediatrics, 1987.
3. Barnhart, S, and Czervinske, MP: Clinical Handbook of Perinatal and Pediatric Respiratory Care. WB Saunders, Philadelphia, 1995, p 267.
4. AARC clinical practice guidelines: Transcutaneous blood gas monitoring for neonatal and pediatric patients. Respiratory Care 39(12):1180, 1994.
5. AARC clinical practice guidelines: Endotracheal suctioning of mechanically ventilated adults and children with artificial airways. Respiratory Care 38(5):500, 1993.
6. AARC clinical practice guidelines: Neonatal time-triggered, pressure-limited, time-cycled mechanical ventilation. Respiratory Care, 39(8):808, 1994.
7. Whitaker, K: Comprehensive Perinatal and Pediatric Respiratory Care. Delmar, NY, 1992, p 287.
8. AARC clinical practice guidelines: Patient-ventilator system checks. Respiratory Care 37(8):882, 1992.
9. AARC clinical practice guidelines: Ventilator circuit changes. Respiratory Care 39(8):797,1994.
10. AARC clinical practice guidelines: Pulse oximetry. Respiratory Care 36(12):1406, 1991.

11. AARC clinical practice guidelines: Oxygen therapy in the home or extended care facility. Respiratory Care 37(8):918, 1992.
12. AARC clinical practice guidelines: Capillary blood gas sampling for neonatal and pediatric patients. Respiratory Care 39(12):1180, 1994.

EXPERT OPINIONS FOR CHAPTER 19

1. Analysis of patient data provides the following interpretations:

    The patient is at...   high risk for airway obstruction due to potential for airway edema
    high risk for oxygenation failure due to potential for carbon monoxide inhalation
    high risk for ventilatory failure due to hypoxemia, lack of ventilatory drive, airway
    obstruction, chest wall restriction, or muscle fatigue
    high risk for infection due to burns, indwelling lines, and physiologic stress

2. Monitoring plan:

    Respiratory-   ABG, co-oximetry, pulmonary mechanics, vital signs, physical observation, capnography, hemodynamics, oxgenation/ventilation indices and criteria (i.e., PaO_2/FiO_2 ratio)

    Cardiovascular-   ECG, vital signs, hemodynamics, physical observation, electrolyte analysis

    Renal-   Urine output, blood urea nitrogen test, creatinine levels, physical observation, skin turgor

    Immune-   White blood counts, cultures, sensitivity tests, temperature

    Integumentary-   Physical observation, skin turgor, wound condition

3. The central venous catheter may be used to monitor fluid status and measure right atrial pressure. In some instances it may reflect other cardiac pressures as well. It may also be used to administer nutritional supplements.

4. The flexible fiberoptic bronchoscope may be of help in intubation when the endotracheal tube is slipped over the FFB tubing. The scope is then used to locate the proper intubation site (i.e., trachea) and the endotracheal tube is passed over the FFB tube and into place in the trachea.

5. Oxygenation status may be evaluated by PO_2, SO_2, AaO_2, PaO_2/PAO_2, PaO_2/FiO_2, Qs/Qt, oxygen content, and physical observation.

6. Strict isolation techniques should be instituted to protect the patient at high risk of infection. Good handwashing is essential.

7. Yes.

8. The oximetry and co-oximetry values differ due to the specific entities measured by each test. Oximeters *do not* differentiate as to what substance is attached to the hemoglobin, but co-oximetry specifically looks at carbon monoxide attached to the hemoglobin. Thus co-oximetry makes a distinction that oximetry does not. Oximeters tend to read falsely high in the presence of carbon monoxide inhalation.

9. Ms. Hayes sodium level is low and her urine output is on the low side of normal. Diastolic blood pressure is also low. Because of the nature of burn injuries, hypovolemia is a likely consequence. These assessments reveal a trend indicating hypovolemia is present.

10. Cloth ties or commercial harness devices are methods of choice when facial burns are present. This negates the need for using adhesive materials on or near burn injuries.

11. $AaO_2 = PAO_2 - PaO_2$
    $PAO_2 = FiO_2 (PB - PH_2O) - PaCO_2$
    $PAO_2 = 1 (760 - 47) - 50$
    $\quad = 663$ mmHg.

    $AaO_2 = 663 - 128$
    $AaO_2 = 535$

12. $CaO_2 = [Hbg. \times 1.34 \times SaO_2] + (PaO_2 \times .003)$
    $CaO_2 = [12 \times 1.34 \times .50] + (128 \times .003)$
    $\quad = 8.04 + .384$
    $\quad = 8.424$ vol %

13. The alveolar-arterial gradient is quite high, indicating poor oxygen exchange. The oxygen content of the arterial blood is normally 20 volume %. The value of 8.424 is very low, indicating poor oxygenation as well.

14. Hyperbaric oxygen therapy may be of help in this case.

15. The associated risks of transporting Ms. Hayes (ventilatory compromise, cardiac disturbance, pain, anxiety) are certainly significant and present. At the same time the benefit of transport must be assessed in light of the potential for improvement in outcome. Transport to a hyperbaric chamber could significantly improve Ms. Hayes oxygenation status.

16. Hyperbaric therapy is " the therapeutic use of oxygen at pressures greater than one atmosphere." Outcomes of hyperbaric therapy include, bubble reduction (air emboli...), increase in tissue oxygenation, vasoconstriction, enhancement of immune function, and neovascularization.[1]

17. The capnograph represents a $PETCO_2$ of 35 mmHg.

18. Proper placement is supported by this data, although more extensive assessment is warranted.

19. Strategies for airway care include scrutinous cuff maintenance or use of a lanz tube or foam cuff.

20. Atrial fibrillation with a ventricular rate of 110 is shown.

21. Intervention may occur using calcium channel blockers or beta blockers.

22. Cardioversion may be indicated if symptoms worsen.

23. Ms. Hayes is improving, as evidenced by the occurrence of normal sinus rhythm and increased levels of cognitive performance.

24 and 25.

Objectives	Interventions	Outcome Evaluations
Maintain airway patency	Secure endotracheal tube Continue airway care	Auscultation of breath sounds and capnography No detection of tidal volume leaks/no tracheal trauma
Assure oxygenation	Supplemental oxygen and/or positive airway pressure	Normal ABG, oximetry, vital signs, oxygen indices
Assure ventilation	PPV as needed Wean as indicated	Normal ABG, breath sounds
Maintain fluid balance	Fluid administration Monitor input/output	Normal urine output, electrolytes, laboratory tests

| Prevent infection | Comply with strict isolation precautions | No active infection detected |
| Optimize recovery | Support educational and emotional needs | Subjective satisfaction |

At this time bronchodilator therapy should be instituted.

26. Circumferential eschars, the crusts or scabs over a burn wound, may restrict the patient's chest expansion, thus adversely effecting ventilation.[2]

27. Pulmonary compliance is worsening. This may be associated with restriction from eschars or some consolidation process within the lung.

28. Aggressive pulmonary hygiene measures should be instituted to promote pulmonary aeration and secretion clearance.

29. Earlier intervention with pulmonary hygiene may indeed have been wise.

30. A side-lying position with head lowered should be used. The patient should lie on her right side to drain the lower left lateral segment.

31. The patient's potassium level is slightly low and should be optimized. In assessing the case so far it should be evident that nutritional requirements should be carefully assessed and optimized as well. The process of burn healing requires a significant increase in daily nutritional requirements.

32. Metabolic calorimetry may be instituted to monitor nutritional status.

33. Weaning plan:

Objectives	Interventions	Outcome Evaluations
Discontinue mechanical ventilatory support	Incremental decrease in ventilatory support using SIMV with PSV as needed.	Maintenance of oxygenation, ventilation and acid-base status
Optimize weaning abilities	Nutritional support, emotional support, clear communication/education, physical reconditioning.	Successful discontinuance of MV

34. Useful weaning criteria include:[3]

Measurement	Criterion
Oxygenation	
PaO_2 (torr) (s 40% O.)	> 60
SaO_2 (%) (s 40% O.)	> 90%
PaO_2/Pao, ratio	> 0.35
PaO_2/FiO, ratio	> 200
Qs/Qt (% shunt)	< 20%
Ventilation	
$PaCo_2$ (torr)	< 50
pH	> 7.35
Ventilatory Mechanics	
Respiratory rate (f) (breaths/min)	< 30

Tidal volume (V1) (mL/kg)	> 5
Vital capacity (VC) (mL/kg)	> 10–15
Static compliance (mL/cm H_2O)	> 30–33

Respiratory Muscle Strength

Maximum inspiratory force (MIF) (—cm H2O)	> 20–30

Ventilatory Demand

Minute volume (VE) for normal PCO_2, (L/min)	< 1–
Vps/VT (dead space fraction) %	< 0.60

Ventilatory Reserve

Maximum voluntary ventilation (MVV) (L/min)	> 20
	> twice VE

Newer criteria include the rapid shallow breathing index, the oxygen cost of breathing (OCB), the CROP index (compliance, rate, oxygenation, and Pmax), and the weaning index (WI). See reference for more information.

35. The flow-volume loop indicates that a fixed obstruction (? tracheal stenosis) is present.

References

1. Weaver, LK: Hyperbaric treatment of respiratory emergencies. Respiratory Care 37(7):720-734, 1992.
2. Golenberg Klein, D: Management of persons with burns. In Medical Surgical Nursing. Mosby, St. Louis, 1991, p 2170.
3. Scanlan, C: Discontinuing ventilatory support. In Egan's Fundamentals of Respiratory Care, ed 6. Mosby, St. Louis, 1995, p 973.

SAMPLE TEST QUESTIONS

Chapter 1 *Questions* . . . .

1. Which of the following is essential to a problem-based learning (PBL) system?
   - I. A well-formulated problem
   - II. Group discussions
   - III. A guided investigation
   - IV. Analytical or inquisitive activities
   - V. An ill-structured problem

   a. I, II, and IV only
   b. III, IV, and V only
   c. II, IV, and V only
   d. I, III, and IV only

2. PBL learning systems are most effective in teaching students:
   a. Basic information
   b. Critical thinking skills
   c. Theories and techniques
   d. Philosophical concepts

3. Drawbacks to the implementation of PBL systems include all of the following EXCEPT:
   a. Resistance to or fear of change on the part of instructors
   b. The active participation of students in the learning process
   c. The lack of available data supporting the effectiveness of PBL
   d. The belief of some that PBL has no long-lasting effect on learning

4. Which of the following is NOT considered an outcome of PBL?
   a. Teacher-centered learning
   b. Lifelong learning
   c. Integration of clinical skills and basic sciences
   d. Problem-solving skills

Use words or phrases from the following list to fill in the blanks in the sentences below.
Note: Do not use any word/phrase more than once; some words/phrases may not be used.

Analysis	Decision making
Application	Integration
Cause and effect diagramming	Information gathering
Concept mapping	Outcomes
Critical thinking	Recall

5. The written examinations offered by the National Board for Respiratory Care (NBRC) involve the elements of _____, _____, and _____.

6. Diagramming an idea to reveal the interrelationships among its parts is called _____.

7. Approaching medical problems from an investigative stance promotes the learning skills of _____ and _____, which are used in the NBRC Clinical Simulation examinations.

8. A useful tool for diagramming the linear relationships of ideas within a concept is the _____.

9. Write a brief paragraph explaining how PBL differs from more traditional teaching/learning styles.

   _____

   _____

   _____

   _____

   _____

   _____

Answers for Chapter 1. . . . .

1. c

2. b

3. b

4. a

5. Recall, application, analysis

6. Concept mapping

7. Information gathering, decision making

8. Cause and effect diagramming

9. The answer should include the following elements: Traditional teaching/learning styles involve passivity on the part of the student, emphasis on recall, and external (teacher-directed) goal setting. PBL promotes active participation on the part of the students, self-setting of goals, problem-solving skills, and critical thinking.

Chapter 2 Questions . . . .

Contrast ordinary thinking and critical thinking by filling in the table with the terms below.

Associating concepts   Evaluating
Assuming   Guessing
Classifying   Supposing

Ordinary Thinking	Critical Thinking
1.	Estimating
Preferring	2.
Grouping	3.
Believing	4.
5.	Grasping Principles
6.	Hypothesizing

7. **Practice strategies for critical thinking include:**
    I.   Self-analysis
    II. Literature review
    III. Brainstorming
    IV. Diagramming

    a. I and IV only
    b. II and III only
    c. I, II, and III only
    d. I, II, III, and IV

8. **Critical-thinking skills may be assessed using:**
    I.   Outcome measurers
    II   Clinical simulation testing
    III. Computerized simulations
    IV. Multiple-choice testing

    a. I and IV only
    b. II and III only
    c. I, II, and III only
    d. I, II, III, and IV

9. **Which of the following would constitute pitfalls or roadblocks to critical thinking?**
    I.   Aggression
    II. Expectancies
    III. Subjectivity
    IV. Metacognition

    a. I and III only
    b. II and IV only
    c. I, II, and III only
    d. I, II, III, and IV

10. **Compared to an expert, a novice is more likely to:**

    I. Depend on memory
    II. Recognize patterns
    III. Use trial and error
    IV. Depend on rules

    a. I, II, and III only
    b. I, III, and IV only
    c. II, III, and IV only
    d. I, II, and IV only

Answers for Chapter 2. . . . .

Ordinary Thinking	Critical Thinking
1. Guessing	Estimating
Preferring	2. Evaluating
Grouping	3. Classifying
Believing	4. Assuming
5. Associating Concepts	Grasping Principles
6. Supposing	Hypothesizing

7. d   9. c

8. d   10. b

Chapter 3 *Questions* . . . .

1. **Which of the following approaches would lead to the most effective patient assessment?**
   a. Assessing every patient in exactly the same way.
   b. Selecting one assessment system and not deviating from it.
   c. Relying totally on your own knowledge and skill.
   d. Modifying assessment technique based on findings.

2. **A good assessment process would involve:**
   I. Detection of unusual events
   II. The use of multiple resources
   III. Good communication skills
   IV. Making a rapid judgment
   V. Establishing and maintaining a systematic approach

   a. I, II, III, and V only
   b. II, III, IV, and V only
   c. I, II, III, and IV only
   d. I, II, III, IV, and V

3. **In a patient assessment by an RCP, information from which of the following sources should be included?**
   I. The patient's medical history
   II. Shift report received from another RCP
   III. A medical dictionary
   IV. Statements from the patient's family or significant other
   V. Results from a cardiac stress test

   a. I, II, III, IV, and V
   b. III, IV, and V only
   c. I, III, and V only
   d. I, II, and IV only

4. **When assessing a patient, a novice, as compared to an expert, is more likely to:**
   I. Depend on memory
   II. Recognize patterns
   III. Use trial and error
   IV. Depend on rules

   a. I, II, and III only
   b. I, III, and IV only
   c. II, III, and IV only
   d. I, II, and IV only

5. **A patient's ability to cooperate during the assessment process would be decreased by:**
   I. Decreased visual acuity
   II. Language barrier
   III. Effects of medication

a. III only
b. I and II only
c. II and III only
d. I, II, and III

6. **When an RCP asks a patient what day of the week it is and in which hospital he or she is, what is being assessed?**
   a. Verbal communication skills
   b. Orientation to time and place
   c. Willingness to cooperate
   d. Emotional stability

7. **A patient's ability to follow instructions would be best indicated by the patient's:**
   a. Being aware of what time it is
   b. Ability to feed herself or himself
   c. Orientation to time and place
   d. Performance of tasks on command

8. **In the assessment of special populations of adults (home care patients, geriatric patients, multicultural settings), major considerations include:**
   I. Assuring that the patient understands the assessor
   II. Paying extra attention to nonverbal clues
   III. Assessing the environment as well as the patient
   IV. Assessing all patients according to the same norms

   a. I, II, and III only
   b. I, II, and IV only
   c. II, III, and IV only
   d. I, III, and IV only

9. **Which of the following are true regarding the assessment of neonatal or pediatric patients?**
   I. Age-appropriate language must be used.
   II. Developmental factors must be considered.
   III. Pediatric norms are essentially scaled down adult norms.
   IV. Assessment techniques must be tailored for the individual patient.

   a. I and II only
   b. I, III, and IV only
   c. I, II, and IV only
   d. II and IV only

10. **The therapeutic objective of an intervention may be said to have been met when:**
    a. The physician discontinues the therapy.
    b. Assessment results no longer indicate the intervention will benefit the patient.
    c. The patient states that the intervention is no longer needed.
    d. All of the above.

Short essay questions

11. **Briefly explain the value of a systematic approach to assessment**

_____

_____

_____

_____

12. List and briefly explain five approaches to a systematic assessment system

_____

_____

_____

_____

_____

Answers for Chapter 3 . . . .

1. d
2. a
3. a
4. b
5. d
6. b
7. d
8. a
9. c
10. b
11. Points to be included in the response include:
    - It allows collection of data in all essential areas.
    - It promotes consistency.
    - It reduces the risk of overlooking significant findings.
12. Approaches listed in the text include:
    - Head-to-toe (or toe-to-head) approach—performing assessment as the body appears.
    - Systems approach—assessing each of the body's systems.
    - Chronological approach—either beginning with earliest symptom/sign or the most recent, assess patient according to the time symptoms/signs appeared.
    - Assessing by exception—assessing unusual events, as unexpected reactions to treatment.
    - Checklist approach—using a prepared list and indicating which items do or do not apply to a patient.
    - Treatment assessments—monitoring a set of parameters associated with a particular treatment or procedure.
    - Systematic pulmonary assessment—assessing for signs/symptoms specifically associated with function of the pulmonary system.

Chapter 4 Questions . . . .

Match the terms in Column B with the terms/phrases in Column A.

		Column A	Column B
____	1.	A focused inquiry	A. Evaluation
____	2.	The use of an appropriate instrument	B. Formative
____	3.	Repeatability of a measurement	C. Impact
____	4.	End product of a process	D. Outcome
____	5.	Ongoing activities	E. Process
____	6.	Effectiveness of a response	F. Reliability
____	7.	An ongoing evaluation	G. Summative
____	8.	End-point evaluation	H. Validity

9. **Which of the following types of instruments could be used to evaluate RCP performance?**
   - I. Peer review
   - II. Employee performance appraisal
   - III. Self-evaluation
   - IV. Competency evaluation
   - V. Client survey

   a. I, III, IV, and V only
   b. II, III, IV, and V only
   c. I, II, III, and IV only
   d. I, II, III, IV, and V

10. **The responsibility for ongoing evaluation systems rests with**
    a. the institutional administration
    b. the RC department management
    c. the CQI committee
    d. all RC personnel

11. **An overall evaluation system for RC would involve:**
    I. Evaluating the patient
    II. Evaluating RCP performance
    III. Evaluating department operation procedures
    IV. Evaluating each piece of RC equipment

    a. II and III only
    b. III and IV only
    c. I and IV only
    d. I, II, III, and IV

12. **Established standards used in respiratory care might include:**
    I. AARC Clinical Practice Guidelines
    II. Results of the NBRC Job Analysis study
    III. NFPA recommendations

    a. I, II, and III
    b. II and III only
    c. I and III only
    d. I and II only

13. **Which of the following is NOT a part of outcome management?**
    a. Setting objectives
    b. Determining blame for errors
    c. Monitoring the evaluation process
    d. Measuring the outcome of the process

Answers for Chapter 4. . . . .

1. a
2. h
3. f
4. d
5. e
6. c
7. b

8. g
9. d
10. d
11. d
12. a
13. b

Chapter 5 *Questions* . . . .

1. **Which of the following is NOT a part of a respiratory care plan?**
    a. Identifies the patient problem
    b. Creates therapeutic objectives
    c. Establishes a decision tree
    d. Provides for continuous regulation

2. **Respiratory care protocols may be oriented toward:**
    I.   Modalities, treatments, or therapies
    II. Patient diseases or conditions
    III. Anticipated patient outcomes

    a. I and II only
    b. II and III only
    c. I and III only
    d. I, II, and III

Use the following information for questions 3 and 4: A 73-year-old man with a longstanding diagnosis of chronic lung disease is being discharged from an acute care setting to a home care setting. He is currently receiving oxygen at 1.5 liters per minute by nasal cannula. His physician requests a recommendation from the RCP.

3. **What should the RCP's first action be?**
    a. Recommend oxygen at home.
    b. Establish therapeutic objectives.
    c. Perform an assessment on the patient.
    d. Develop an intervention plan.

4. **The patient is to receive oxygen at home using an oxygen concentrator. What should the RCP's next action be?**
    a. Instruct patient on safety aspects associated with oxygen concentrators.
    b. Develop a plan for continued monitoring of the patient.
    c. Establish therapeutic objectives.
    d. Make recommendations for the adjustment of the therapy in the new setting.

5. **An RC protocol must contain at least which of the following elements?**
    I.   Clearly stated objectives
    II   Date on which the protocol is to be discontinued
    III. A decision tree or algorithm
    IV. Potential complications
    V.   Decision points where physician must be contacted

    a. I, II, III, IV, and V
    b. I, II, IV, and V only
    c. I, III, IV, and V only
    d. II, III, and V only

6. **Which of the following are acceptable indications for modifying an RC plan?**
   I. Time restrictions
   II. Incorrect initial choice for intervention
   III. Lack of compliance on the part of the patient
   IV. Changes in the patient's condition

   a. II and IV only
   b. II, III, and IV only
   c. I, II, and IV only
   d. I, II, III, and IV

7. **Briefly explain the purpose of a respiratory care plan.**

   _____

   _____

   _____

   _____

   _____

   _____

8. **How is each of the following critical-thinking skills used in the development of a respiratory care plan?**
   a. Analysis
   b. Evaluation
   c. Inference
   d. Self-regulation

Answers for Chapter 5. . . . .

1. c

2. a

3. b

4. c

5. c

6. d

7. The answer should include the following elements: to deliver high-quality care to the patient, to encompass the needs of the patient, and to encompass the potential outcomes of a particular intervention.

8. Student should be able to explain that each critical-thinking skill listed is used in each step of developing a respiratory care plan.

Chapter 6 *Questions* . . . .

1–6: Which of the following activities promote:

> A. Good time management
> B. Poor time management

___ 1. Arranging priorities based on importance of the task

___ 2. Performing short-time tasks first.

___ 3. Performing least interesting tasks at peak energy times.

___ 4. Analyzing each task continually

___ 5. Delegating appropriate tasks.

___ 6. Always working at "top speed."

7. If two tasks are scheduled to be performed at the same time, the RCP should:
   a. Delegate one task to another person.
   b. Perform tasks in the order in which they were received.
   c. Prioritize the tasks before making a decision.
   d. Complete the task that requires the least time first.

8. Once a time-management path has been mapped out:
   > I. It should be followed without deviation.
   > II. It may require modification based on subsequent events.
   > III. It should be constantly reevaluated.

   a. I and II only
   b. II and III only
   c. I and III only
   d. I, II, and III

9. Which of the following are tools that may be used in effective time management?
   > I. Check lists for documentation of therapy and patient assessment
   > II. Priority or triage scoring systems
   > III. Flexible staff scheduling

   a. I and III only
   b. II and III only
   c. I and II only
   d. I, II, and III

10. Giving purpose and order to the allocation of time is called
_____.

11. Possibly the key characteristic enabling an individual to use good time management
is _____.

12. Comparing the amount of time required to perform a task to the Uniform Reporting
Manual is one way to measure _____.

13. Comparing the level of achievement actually reached to the original goal is a method
of measuring _____.

14. Negative outcomes related to lack of time structure include (list at least 4):

_____

_____

_____

_____

Answers for Chapter 6. . . . .

1. a
2. b
3. a
4. b
5. a
6. b
7. c

8. b
9. d
10. Time structure
11. Self-discipline
12. Efficiency
13. Effectiveness
14. Depression, psychological distress, anxiety, neuroticism, physical symptoms, hopelessness, and so on.

Chapter 7 *Questions* . . . .

Use the following information for questions 1–15: Mr. Tie is a 33-year-old accountant with a 36 pack-year history of cigarette smoking. He is 75 inches (190 cm) tall and weighs 190 pounds (80 kg) and exercises regularly. He is scheduled for a right–upper-lobe lobectomy.

Indicate which of the following would be (+) and would NOT be (0) risk factors for postoperative complications on this patient.

____   1.   The nature of the surgery

____   2.   The patient's age

____   3.   The patient's smoking history

____   4.   The patient's occupation

____   5.   The patient's general physical condition

____   6.   The patient's weight

____   7.   The use of general anesthesia

Indicate which of the following would be (+) and would NOT be (0) anticipated respiratory concerns postoperatively for this patient.

____   8.   Atelectasis

____   9.   Hypoxemia

____   10.   Secretion retention

____   11.   Hypoventilation

____   12.   Bronchospasm

____   13.   Hypercapnea

____   14.   Ineffective cough

____   15.   Increased functional residual capacity (FRC)

Indicate which of the monitoring/assessment techniques in Column B would be used to assess whether each of the possible complications listed in Column A is present. NOTE: Multiple techniques may be used to detect some complications. Some of the monitoring/assessment techniques may be used more than once; some may not be used at all.

_____ 16. Atelectasis   A. Inspection

_____ 17. Hypoxemia   B. Palpation

_____ 18. Secretion retention   C. Percussion

_____ 19. Hypoventilation   D. Auscultation

_____ 20. Bronchospasm   E. Pulse oximetry

_____ 21. Hypercapnea   F. Arterial blood gas analysis (ABG)

_____ 22. Ineffective cough   G. Peak flow (PF)

                                   H. Complete pulmonary function test (PFT)

                                   I. Chest X-ray (CXR)

                                   J. Body temperature

23. The definition of atelectasis is _____.

24. In addition to turning, coughing, and deep breathing, the most common intervention used to treat postoperative atelectasis is _____.

25. Atelectasis may cause an increase in the work of breathing to a(n) (increase/decrease) in pulmonary compliance.

26. In the presence of atelectasis, hypoxemia may occur owing to _____.

27. Therapeutic objectives for oxygen administration postoperatively might include:
    I.   Maintain PaO_2 between 80 and 100 mm Hg
    II. Maintain SaO_2 greater than 92%
    III. Increase lung compliance to 100 mL/cm H_2O
    IV. Decrease work of breathing

    a. I and II only
    b. I, II, and III only
    c. I, II, III, and IV
    d. none of the objectives listed

28. **Therapeutic interventions for secretion removal on a postoperative patient might include turning, coughing, deep breathing, and which of the following?**

      I.   Intermittent positive pressure breathing (IPPB)
      II. Chest physiotherapy (CPT) and postural drainage (PD)
      III. Nasotracheal suctioning
      IV. Continuous positive airway pressure (CPAP)

    a. I, II, and III only
    b. II, III, and IV only
    c. II and III only
    d. I, II, III, and IV

Answers for Chapter 7. . . . .

1. Yes (+)
2. No (0)
3. Yes (+)
4. No (0)
5. No (0)
6. No (0)
7. Yes(+)
8. Yes (+)
9. Yes (+)
10. Yes (+)
11. Yes (+)
12. No (0)
13. Yes (+)
14. Yes (+)
15. No (0)

16. a, b, c, d, j
17. e, f
18. d
19. f
20. d, g (not h; complete pulmonary function tests would not be done on a postoperative patient)
21. f
22. a, d
23. An airless condition of the alveoli; or a collapsed region of the lung
24. Incentive spirometry
25. Decrease
26. V/Q mismatch or intrapulmonary shunting
27. a
28. c

Chapter 8 *Questions* . . . .

1. Other than wheezing, common presenting factors for children with an acute asthmatic episode include:
    - I.   Nonproductive cough
    - II. Tachycardia
    - III. Fever
    - IV. *Pulsus paradoxus*

    - a. I, II, and III only
    - b. I, III, and IV only
    - c. II and IV only
    - d. I, II, III, and IV

2. Frequently, laboratory assessment of children with an acute asthmatic episode reveals:
    - I.   Hypoxemia
    - II. Hypercapnea
    - III. Eosinophilia
    - IV. Peak flow <40% of predicted

    - a. I, II, and IV only
    - b. I, III, and IV only
    - c. I and II only
    - d. I, II, III, and IV

3. Asthma is classified as:
    - a. A restrictive disease
    - b. An obstructive disease
    - c. An infectious disease
    - d. A neoplastic disorder

4. The primary feature of asthma is:
    - a. Mucosal edema
    - b. Irreversible bronchoconstriction
    - c. Reversible bronchoconstriction
    - d. Pulmonary consolidation

5. Precipitating factors for an acute asthma episode include:
    - I.   Respiratory infections
    - II. Specific allergens
    - III. Exercise
    - IV. Emotional distress

    - a. I and II only
    - b. I, II, and III only
    - c. II, III, and IV only
    - d. I, II, III, and IV

6–15: Indicate which of the following would (+) and would NOT (0) commonly be included in the initial treatment of an acute asthmatic episode.

____   6.   Oxygen

____   7. β_2 adrenergic aerosol

____   8.   Corticosteroids

____   9.   Antibiotics

____   10.   Cromolyn sodium aerosol

____   11.   Parasympatholytic aerosol

____   12.   Endotracheal intubation and mechanical ventilation

____   13.   Methyl xanthines

____   14.   Sedatives or narcotics

____   15.   Mucolytic aerosol (e.g., acetyl cysteine)

16–21: Indicate which of the following would (+) and would NOT (0) commonly be included in patient/parent education for an asthmatic child.

____   16.   Appropriate use of a peak flow meter

____   17.   Symptom recognition

____   18.   Monitoring for allergens

____   19.   Appropriate use of incentive spirometry

____   20.   Appropriate use of pulse oximetry

____   21.   Appropriate use of metered dose inhalers (MDI)

Answers for Chapter 8. . . . .

1. b
2. b
3. b
4. c
5. d
6. Yes (+)
7. Yes (+)
8. Yes (+)
9. No (0)
10. No (0)
11. Yes(+)

12. No (0)
13. Yes(+)
14. No (0)
15. No (0)
16. Yes(+)
17. Yes (+)
18. Yes (+)
19. No (0)
20. No (0)
21. Yes(+)

Chapter 9 *Questions* . . . .

1–7: Indicate which of the following would (+) and would NOT (0) be an indication for fiberoptic bronchoscopy.

____   1.   To investigate the presence of lesions of unknown etiology which are noted on X-ray.

____   2.   To remove a foreign body.

____   3.   To obtain lower respiratory tract secretions.

____   4.   To aid in routine intubations.

____   5.   To investigate lesions of the nasal passages, pharynx, and larynx.

____   6.   To remove mucus plugs responsible for lobar or segmental atelectasis.

____   7.   To obtain tissue specimens from the lung parenchyma.

8. The effect of the human immunovirus (HIV) on the lungs is:
   a. It causes an acute bronchiolitis.
   b. It creates pulmonary consolidation and pneumonia.
   c. It allows for opportunistic infections to develop.
   d. It is a causative agent for pulmonary neoplasms.

9. A CD4 lymphocyte count of less than 200 is indicative of:
   a. Immunosuppression
   b. Wide spread infection
   c. Successful antibiotic therapy
   d. A neoplastic process

10. Pulmonary infections commonly associated with AIDS include:
   I. Mycobacterium tuberculosis
   II. Pneumocystis carinii
   III. Candida albicans

   a. II only
   b. I and II only
   c. I and III only
   d. I, II, and III

11. Drugs commonly used to treat tuberculosis include:
   I. Isoniazid
   II. Ethanbutol

    III. Amphotericin B
    IV. Rifampin

  a. I, II, and III only
  b. II, III, and IV only
  c. I, II, and IV only
  d. I, II, III, and IV

12. **HIV attacks which of the following blood cells?**
  a. Erythrocytes
  b. Lymphocytes
  c. Basophils
  d. Eosinophils

13. **Which of the following is NOT a type of T-lymphocyte?**
  a. Helper T-lymphocyte
  b. Killer T-lymphocyte
  c. Suppresser T-lymphocyte
  d. Phagocytic T-lymphocyte

14. **Which of the following drugs is commonly used to treat pneumocystic infections?**
  a. Ribavirin
  b. Polymyxin B
  c. Pentamidine
  d. Erythromycin

15. **Universal precautions are used in health-care settings to protect:**
  a. Patients from acquiring microbes from health-care staff.
  b. Health-care staff from acquiring microbes from patients.
  c. Health-care staff from acquiring microbes from each other.
  d. All of the above

16. **The single most important aspect of universal precautions involves:**
  a. Good handwashing practices.
  b. Gloves, gowns, and other barrier devices.
  c. Avoiding direct contact with infected patients.
  d. Avoiding sharp instruments (needles, scalpels, etc.)

17. **Having patients rinse their mouth or gargle before a sputum induction procedure is done to:**
  a. Anesthetize the oral cavity and upper airway.
  b. Remove unpleasant tasting medication residues form the mouth.
  c. Decrease the chance of a contaminated specimen.
  d. All of the above.

18. **Responsibilities of the RCP in the treatment of patients with AIDS include:**
    I. Providing knowledgeable and skillful treatment.
    II. Providing emotional support for the patients and their families.
    III. Acting as a resource for other health-care practitioners.
    IV. Deferring to the physician on all aspects of care.

  a. I and III only
  b. II, III, and IV only

c. I, II, and III only
d. I, II, III, and IV

Answers for Chapter 9. . . . .

1. Yes (+)
2. Yes (+)
3. Yes (+)
4. No (0)
5. No (0)
6. Yes (+)
7. No (0)
8. c
9. a

10. d
11. c
12. b
13. d
14. c
15. d
16. a
17. c
18. c

Chapter 10 *Questions* . . . .

1–6: Indicate which of the following would (+) and would NOT (0) be common physical findings in a patient with sleep apnea syndrome (SAS).

____   1.   Obesity

____   2.   A long neck

____   3.   A short jaw (micrognathia)

____   4.   A large tongue (macroglossia)

____   5.   Enlarged tonsils

____   6.   Chronic bronchitis

7–17: Indicate which of the following would (+) and would NOT (0) be common clinical findings in a patient with sleep apnea syndrome (SAS).

____   7.   Increased red blood cell count (RBC)

____   8.   Snoring

____   9.   Daytime sleepiness

____   10.   Chronic hypoxia

____   11.   Chronic hypoventilation

____   12.   Memory loss

____   13.   Increased white blood cell count (WBC)

____   14.   Decreased total lung capacity (TLC)

____   15.   Chronic respiratory alkalosis

____   16.   Cardiac arrhythmias

____   17.   Narcolepsy

18. The intermittent blockage of the upper airway during sleep in the presence of a normal respiratory drive is called _____ sleep apnea.

19. The intermittent absence of respiratory effort during sleep in the presence of a patent airway is called _____ sleep apnea.

20. A third type of sleep apnea is a combination of the other two and is called _____ sleep apnea.

21. The two major stages of sleep are _____ and _____.

22. An elevated level of red blood cells (RBC) is called _____.

23. Insufficient ventilation to meet the body's metabolic needs is called _____.

24. Right ventricular failure due to disorders of the lung is called _____.

25–34: Indicate which of the following would (+) and would NOT (0) be normally recorded while performing a polysomnograph test.

_____   25.   Arterial oxygen saturation

_____   26.   Central venous pressure

_____   27.   Eye movement

_____   28.   Nasal air flow

_____   29.   Electrocardiogram (ECG)

_____   30.   Electroencephalogram (EEG)

_____   31.   Electromylogram (EMG)

_____   32.   Pulmonary artery pressure

_____   33.   Arterial blood gases

_____   34.   Vital capacity

35–41: Indicate which of the following would (+) and would NOT (0) be considered as a part of the treatment plan for a patient with obstructive sleep apnea (OSA).

_____   35.   Weight loss

____ 36. **Sedatives**

____ 37. **Upper airway surgery**

____ 38. **Continuous positive airway pressure (CPAP)**

____ 39. **Bronchodilator therapy**

____ 40. **Tracheotomy**

____ 41. **Oral or dental prosthetic appliances**

42. **Which of the following statements is (are) true concerning the treatment of central sleep apnea (CSA)?**
    I.   Noninvasive positive pressure ventilation (NIPPV) has been of some benefit in some patients
    II. CSA is successfully treated in much the same way as OSA.
    III. There has been no uniformly accepted successful treatment for CSA.

    a. I and II only
    b. I and III only
    c. III only
    d. II only

Answers for Chapter 10 . . . .

1. Yes (+)
2. No (0)
3. Yes (+)
4. Yes (+)
5. Yes (+)
6. No (0)
7. Yes (+)
8. Yes (+)
9. Yes (+)
10. Yes (+)
11. Yes (+)
12. Yes (+)
13. No (0)
14. No (0)
15. No (0)
16. Yes (+)
17. No (0)
18. Obstructive
19. Central
20. Mixed
21. Rapid eye movement (REM) and non-rapid eye movement (NREM)

22. Polycythemia
23. Hypoventilation
24. Cor pulmonale
25. Yes (+)
26. Yes (+)
27. Yes (+)
28. Yes (+)
29. Yes (+)
30. Yes (+)
31. Yes (+)
32. No (0)
33. No (0)
34. No (0)
35. Yes (+)
36. No (0)
37. Yes (+)
38. Yes (+)
39. No (0)
40. Yes (+)
41. Yes (+)
42. b

Chapter 11 *Questions* . . . .

1–8: Indicate which of the following would (+) and would NOT (0) indicate the possibility of Guillain-Barré syndrome.

____   1.   Obesity

____   2.   Fever

____   3.   A history of cigarette smoking

____   4.   A history of recent upper-respiratory infection

____   5.   Progressive ascending muscle weakness

____   6.   Unilateral paresthesia

____   7.   "Droopy" eyelids

____   8.   Elevated protein levels in cerebral spinal fluid (CSF)

9–13: Indicate which of the following would (+) and would NOT (0) be included among the early interventions for a patient with Guillain-Barré syndrome.

____   9.   Corticosteroid administration

____   10.   Anticholinesterase drug administration (e.g., neostigmine)

____   11.   Bronchodilator therapy

____   12.   Close monitoring of ventilatory mechanics

____   13.   Vasopressive drugs

14. The single most important aspect of the treatment of patients with Guillain-Barré syndrome is _____.

15. List the respiratory parameters that should be monitored in a patient with Guillain-Barré syndrome.

_____

_____

16. Briefly explain why frequent monitoring of the respiratory status of patients with Guillain-Barré syndrome is important.

_____

_____

_____

17. List two respiratory complications frequently seen in patients with Guillain Barré syndrome

    a. _____

    b. _____

18. What would be considered a "critical value" for each of the respiratory parameters listed below?

    a. Vital capacity (VC); Critical value = _____

    b. Tidal volume (V_T); Critical value = _____

    c. Maximum inspiratory pressure (MIP) Critical value = _____

Answers for Chapter 11 . . . .

1. No (0)
2. No (0)
3. No (0)
4. Yes (+)
5. Yes (+)
6. No (0)
7. No (0)
8. Yes (+)
9. No (0)
10. No (0)
11. No (0)
12. Yes (+)
13. No (0)
14. Respiratory monitoring and support

15. Primarily vital capacity (VC), tidal volume (V_T), maximum inspiratory pressure (MIP) [also called negative inspiratory force (NIF)]. Also important: Respiratory frequency (f or RR), Oxygen saturation, and arterial blood gas analysis (ABG, including PaO_2, $PaCO_2$, and pH

16. Paralysis of respiratory muscles may occur over a very short period of time.

17. Atelectasis (and associated intrapulmonary shunt and hypoxemia)

    Ineffective cough (and associated secretion retention and respiratory infection)

18. a. 10–12 mL/kg of ideal body weight or two times tidal volume

    b. 5–7 mL/kg of ideal body weight

    c. –20 cm H_2O pressure

Chapter 12 Questions . . . .

1–7: Indicate which of the following is usually associated with:

  A.   Croup (laryngotracheobronchitis [LTB])
  B.   Epiglottitis
  C.   Both croup and epiglottitis

____ 1.   It is of viral origin.

____ 2.   It is of bacterial origin.

____ 3.   It has a sudden, acute onset.

____ 4.   There is an elevated level of white blood cells (WBC) (leukocytosis).

____ 5.   It occurs mostly in children over 3 years old.

____ 6.   It effects the subglottic area.

____ 7.   The patient drools and has difficulty swallowing.

8. Stridor is defined as _____.

9. The drawing of the skin and tissues surrounding the rib cage during inspiration is called _____.

10. In severe croup, blood gas analysis shows a(an) _____ in PaO_2, a(an) _____ in $PaCO_2$, and a(an) _____ in pH.

11. The respiratory treatment of croup frequently includes:
    I. Oxygen administration
    II. Chest physiotherapy and postural drainage
    III. Cool mist aerosols
    IV. Mechanical ventilation

   a. I and III only
   b. II and III only
   c. I, III, and IV only
   d. I, II, III, and IV

12. **The aerosolized drug of choice to treat acute croup is:**
    a. Albuterol
    b. Epinephrine
    c. Terbutaline
    d. Ipratropium

13. **The desired effect of aerosolized drug administration in croup is:**
    a. Bronchodilation
    b. Vasoconstriction
    c. Cardiac stimulation
    d. Analgesia

14. **Croup may develop into a respiratory emergency if:**
    I.   The patient becomes exhausted because of increased work of breathing.
    II. Airway edema causes a total airway obstruction.
    III. Atelectasis develops.

    a. I and II only
    b. II and III only
    c. I and III only
    d. I, II, and III

15. **When a child is being mechanically ventilated, the ventilator should be set to deliver a tidal volume of:**
    a. 5–10 mL/kg of body weight
    b. 10–15 mL/kg of body weight
    c. 7–10 mL/month of age
    d. 7–10 mL/cm H_2O

16. **A 2-year-old child with croup has been mechanically ventilated using an uncuffed endotracheal tube. After the second day a small leak develops around the tube. This is likely to indicate that:**
    a. Reintubation with a larger endotracheal tube is necessary.
    b. The endotracheal tube has slipped too far down into the airway.
    c. The patient requires more frequent suctioning.
    d. Mucosal edema has decreased.

Answers for Chapter 12 . . . .

1. a
2. b
3. b
4. b
5. b
6. a
7. b
8. A harsh, grating breath sound originating in the upper airway

9. Retraction
10. Decrease or drop in PaO_2; an increase or rise in $PaCO_2$; a decrease or drop in pH
11. a
12. b
13. b
14. a
15. b
16. d

Chapter 13 *Questions* . . . .

1. Drowning is death from _____ as a result of submersion.

2. Near-drowning involves successful resuscitation after submersion and survival for a minimum of _____ hours.

3. About 10–15% of drowning victims die from "dry drowning," which is a result of _____.

4. The major clinical problems involved in all near-drowning victims are related to _____ and _____.

5. Although some degree of pulmonary edema seen in near-drowning victims may be accounted for by aspirated water, the majority of edema fluid is a result of _____.

6. Victims who succumb to the delayed effects of submersion are said to have died from _____.

7. In near-drowning victims, pulse and blood pressure are often difficult to detect because of the effects of _____.

8. Metabolic acidosis usually develops in near-drowning victims because of _____.

9. In near-drowning victims, neurologic damage frequently occurs because of _____.

10. Auscultation of a near-drowning victim is likely to reveal _____ and _____.

11. Near-drowning in cold water may actually increase the victim's chance for survival because of _____.

12–21: Match the respiratory/medical concern in Column A with the likely cause in Column B. NOTE: Items in Column A may have more than one likely cause; items in Column B may be used more than once or not at all.

Column A	Column B
____ 12. Bronchospasm	A. Absorption of water

____ 13. Decreased compliance

____ 14. Decreased hemoglobin, and hematocrit

____ 15. Electrolyte abnormalities

____ 16. Hypercapnia

____ 17. Hypoventilation

____ 18. Hypoxemia

____ 19. Increased airway resistance

____ 20. Infection

____ 21. V/Q mismatching

B. Aspiration of debris

C. Consolidation and atelectasis

D. Loss of respiratory drive

E. Loss of surfactant

F. Mucosal edema

22. **During the transport of a mechanically ventilated patient between hospitals, which of the following emergency supplies must be available?**
   I. Self-inflating resuscitation bag and mask
   II. Portable suction unit with supplies
   III. Laryngoscope and other intubation supplies (including ET tubes)
   IV. Portable oxygen source of adequate volume
   V. Tracheotomy tray and supplies

   a. I, III, IV, and V only
   b. I, II, III, and IV only
   c. II, III, IV, and V only
   d. I, II, III, IV, and V

23–30: **During the transport of a mechanically ventilated patient between hospitals, indicate whether each of the following patient parameters should be monitored:**

   A.   **Continuously**
   B.   **Intermittently**
   C.   **Does not need to be monitored during transport**

____ 23. Respiratory rate

____ 24. Tidal volume

____ 25. Airway pressure

____ 26. Arterial blood gases

____ 27. Electrocardiogram (ECG)

____ 28. **Heart rate**

____ 29. **Breath sounds**

____ 30. **Pulse oximetry**

Answers for Chapter 13 . . . .

1. Asphyxiation
2. 24 hours
3. Glottic spasm (laryngospasm)
4. Hypoxia and acidemia
5. Capillary leakage
6. Secondary drowning
7. Vasoconstriction
8. Hypoxia (both circulatory and hypoxic hypoxia)
9. Cerebral ischemia (hypoxia)
10. Wheezes and crackles (rhonchi and rales)
11. Hypothermia (decreased metabolic rate)
12. B
13. C
14. A
15. A

16. D
17. D
18. C
19. B, F
20. B
21. C
22. B
23. B
24. B
25. B
26. C
27. A
28. A
29. B
30. A

Chapter 14 *Questions* . . . .

1. A general precaution associated with the administration of oxygen is to avoid administering high concentrations to patients with known COPD. Under which of the following circumstances does this precaution NOT apply?

   I. Severe hypoxia
   II. Hypocapnea
   III. The patient is being mechanically ventilated

   a. I and II only
   b. I and III only
   c. II and III only
   d. I, II, and III

2. Mechanical ventilation is being initiated on a 65-year-old female patient who is 62 inches tall and weighs 194 pounds (88 kg). Which of the following would be the most appropriate tidal volume and respiratory frequency?

   a. 600 mL; 12 bpm
   b. 750 mL; 14 bpm
   c. 900 mL; 12 bpm
   d. 1000 mL; 10 bpm

3. Which of the following would be considered contraindications to high levels of PEEP?

   I. A patient with elevated intracranial pressure (ICP)
   II. A patient with increased functional residual capacity (FRC)
   III. A hypovolemic patient
   IV. A patient with a reduced cardiac output (CO)

   a. I, II, and III only
   b. II, III, and IV only
   c. I, III, and IV only
   d. I, II, III, and IV

4. Which of the following would NOT be seen in the ECG of a patient with a myocardial infarction?

   a. Inverted P waves
   b. Presence of Q waves
   c. ST elevation in V leads
   d. Wide QRS complexes

5. Which of the following levels of lactate dehydrogenase (LD) and creatine kinase (CK) would be expected 72 hours after an acute myocardial infarction?

   a. LD near peak value; CK near normal
   b. LD rising; CK rising
   c. LD near normal; CK near peak
   d. LD near normal; CK near normal

6.   Hazards associated with thrombolytic therapy in the treatment of acute myocardial infarction include:

 I.   Cranial hemorrhage
 II. Allergic reactions
 III. Prolonged bleeding time

a.   I and II only
b.   II and III only
c.   I and III only
d.   I, II, and III

7–14:   After increasing the level of PEEP on a mechanically ventilated patient, the following changes were noted. Indicate which of them would be benign or potentially helpful to the patient (+) and which would be potentially harmful (0).

_____   7.   **Increased intracranial pressure (ICP)**

_____   8.   **Increased static compliance**

_____   9.   **Increased arteriovenous oxygen content difference**

_____   10. **Increased PaO$_2$**

_____   11. **Increased pulmonary capillary wedge pressure (PCWP)**

_____   12. **Decreased PvO$_2$**

_____   13. **Decreased oxygen delivery**

_____   14. **Decreased cardiac output (CO)**

Answers for Chapter 14 . . . .

1. d
2. a
3. d
4. a
5. a
6. d
7. Harmful (0)

8. Helpful (+)
9. Harmful (0)
10. Helpful (+)
11. Harmful (0)
12. Harmful (0)
13. Harmful (0)
14. Harmful (0)

Chapter 15 *Questions* . . . .

1. Oxygen therapy is indicated for home use when the patient's PaO_2 is _____ or the saturation is _____.

2. In the evaluation of hypoxemia/desaturation during exercise, a decrease of _____%, as measured by pulse oximetry or _____%, as measured by co-oximetry is considered significant.

3. Prevention of nocturnal hypoventilation and desaturation, improved daytime blood gases and lung volumes, and avoidance of the necessity for tracheostomy have all been claimed as beneficial effects of _____ _____.

4. COPD is an acronym for _____.

5. The majority of COPD patients have a combination of the respiratory diseases _____ and _____.

6. The one etiologic factor that most COPD patients have in common is _____.

7. The general goal for the management of COPD is _____ _____.

8. A liquid oxygen cylinder holding 1 kg (2.2 lb) of liquid will provide about _____ liters of oxygen gas.

9–15: Taking into account convenience, expense, and safety, for each situation below select the most appropriate home oxygen supply source.

9. The patient requires continuous oxygen at 2 lpm (tank/concentrator)

10. The patient requires oxygen at 1 lpm for 6–8 hours per day. (liquid/concentrator)

11. The patient requires frequent oxygen at 1 lpm but likes to work in the garden. (small cylinder/concentrator)

12. The patient lives in an area that has frequent power outages. (liquid/concentrator)

13. The patient requires a continuous aerosol with 30% oxygen at night. (cylinder/liquid)

14. **The patient has a small house heated with a kerosene heater. (liquid/concentrator)**

15. **The patient makes frequent trips to church, shopping, etc. (liquid/concentrator)**

Answers for Chapter 15 . . . .

1. PaO_2 <55 mm Hg; saturation <88%

2. 4%; 2%

3. Noninvasive positive pressure ventilation (NIPPV)

4. Chronic obstructive pulmonary disease

5. Chronic bronchitis and emphysema

6. Cigarette smoking

7. To slow the progression of the disease

8. 700 liters (1000 g/32 g/mole) $\times$ 22.4 L/mole)

9. Concentrator

10. Concentrator

11. Small cylinder

12. Liquid

13. Cylinder

14. Concentrator

15. Liquid

Chapter 16 *Questions* . . . .

1. Which of the following are indicators for the initiation of cardiopulmonary resuscitation?

    I.   Life-threatening dysrhythmias
    II. Acute myocardial infarction with cardiodynamic instability
    III. Anaphylaxis
    IV. Spinal cord injury

    a. I, II, and III only
    b. II, III, and IV only
    c. I, II, and IV only
    d. I, II, III, and IV

2. Hazards associated with cardiopulmonary resuscitation include:

    I.   Cervical spine trauma
    II. Aspiration
    III. Hyperventilation
    IV. Induction of malignant dysrhythmias
    V.   Cardiac tamponade

    a. I, II, and III only
    b. II, IV, and V only
    c. III, IV, and V only
    d. I, II, III, IV, and V

3. A fracture of three or more ribs in two or more places is called:
    a. Pendelluft
    b. Osteothorax
    c. Flail chest
    d. Paradoxical chest

4. An RCP is performing cardiopulmonary resuscitation and notes that the patient's trachea is shifted to the right and that it is becoming increasingly more difficult to ventilate him. In addition, the victim's color is becoming progressively worse, and the carotid pulse is weak on cardiac compression. The patient most likely is suffering from:
    a. Flail chest
    b. Cardiac tamponade
    c. Pneumothorax
    d. Right mainstem bronchial intubation

5. If a pneumothorax is suspected, the most important diagnostic procedure would be:
    a. Vital capacity
    b. Arterial blood gases
    c. Chest X-ray
    d. Maximum inspiratory force

6. **If right mainstem intubation is suspected, the RCP should:**
    a. Request a chest X-ray
    b. Withdraw the endotracheal tube about 2 cm
    c. Request that a tracheotomy be performed
    d. Decrease the tidal volume the patient is receiving

7. **Which of the following is true concerning the management of traumatic head injuries?**
    I.   Mechanical ventilation is required for patients with a Glasgow Coma Scale score of <7.
    II. Mechanical hyperventilation may help to decrease cerebral swelling.
    III. Even short-term ischemia may exacerbate the injury.
    IV. Intercranial pressure should be maintained under 20 mm Hg.

    a. I, II, III, and IV
    b. I, II, and III only
    c. II, III, and IV only
    d. II and III only

8. **After repositioning a patient in bed, it is noticed that the transducer for the pulmonary artery line is approximately 6 in (15 cm) higher than the patient's thorax. How would this affect the readings being made?**
    a. The readings would continue to be accurate.
    b. The readings would be too high.
    c. The readings would be too low.
    d. The effect on the readings would depend on the type and brand of the transducer.

9. **Which of the following is true concerning patient-ventilatory system checks?**
    I.   They must involve observations of the ventilator settings at the time of the check.
    II. They must be ordered by the physician.
    III. They must include documentation of measured patient parameters at the time of the check.
    IV. They must include documentation of the practitioner's observations of the patient at the time of the check.

    a. I, II, III, and IV
    b. I, II, and III only
    c. I, III, and IV only
    d. II, III, and IV only

10. **A severe, high cervical (above C-3) injury will result in:**
    a. The death of the victim
    b. Loss or decrease in cerebral function
    c. Loss of respiratory muscle function
    d. Loss of intercostal muscle but maintenance of diaphragmatic control

11. **Which of the following standards must be met before a patient is considered a good candidate for home ventilatory support?**
    I.   Absence of severe dyspnea while on a ventilator
    II. Inspired oxygen concentrations that are relatively low
    III. Psychological stability
    IV. A stable oral or nasal endotracheal tube

    a. I, II, and III only
    b. II, III, and IV only
    c. I, II, and IV only
    d. I, II, III, and IV

12. **Minimum available alarms on a home care ventilator include:**
    I.   Power failure
    II. Loss of gas source
    III. Exhalation valve failure
    IV. Loss of PEEP

    a. I, II, and III only
    b. II, III, and IV only
    c. I, II, and IV only
    d. I, II, III, and IV

13. **Which of the following items is NOT included on the Glascow Coma Scale?**
    a. Motor response
    b. Verbal response
    c. Eye opening
    d. Respiratory effort

Answers for Chapter 16 . . . .

1. d   8. c
2. d   9. c
3. c   10. c
4. c   11. a
5. c   12. a
6. b   13. d
7. a

Chapter 17 Questions . . . .

1. An Apgar score is used to determine _____.

2. A Dubowitz score is used to determine _____.

3. The primary rationale for the administration of nitric oxide is:
   a. It acts as an analgesic/anesthetic.
   b. It acts as a pulmonary vasodilator.
   c. It acts as a coronary vasodilator.
   d. It prevents the development of methemoglobinemia.

4. Meconium is:
   a. Normally found in the neonate's intestine.
   b. Normally found in amniotic fluid.
   c. Secreted by the placenta.
   d. A result of intrauterine pathology.

5. Meconium aspiration is most commonly associated with:
   I.   Premature infants
   II. Postterm infants
   III. Fetal distress

   a. I and III only
   b. II and III only
   c. I only
   d. III only

6. Which is NOT a common finding in neonates with meconium aspiration?
   a. Lecithin/sphingomyelin ratio less than 2:1
   b. Increased AP diameter of chest
   c. Hypoxia
   d. Mixed acidosis

7. Meconium stained infants should be suctioned:
   a. As soon as the head has been delivered.
   b. After the chest has been delivered.
   c. Immediately after delivery is complete.
   d. Not until after tracheal intubation has been accomplished.

8. Which of the following treatments is likely to be effective in treating meconium aspiration?
   I.   Maintain high PaO_2
   II. Chest physiotherapy and postural drainage during first 8 hours.
   III. Maintain ventilation with high inspiratory times.

   a. I and II only
   b. II and III only

c. I and III only
d. I, II, and III

9. **Which of the following complications are associated with meconium aspiration?**
    I.   Airway inflammation
    II. "Ball-valve" obstruction of small airways
    III. Pneumothorax
    IV. Hyperinflation of some areas of the lungs

    a. I, II, and III only
    b. II, III, and IV only
    c. I, III, and IV only
    d. I, II, III, and IV

10. **One advantage of high frequency ventilation of the neonate is:**
    a. Lower mean airway pressures may be used.
    b. The equipment is easier to use than traditional ventilators.
    c. It does not require endotracheal intubation.
    d. It provides for an increased time constant.

11. **Pneumothorax in the neonate is most effectively diagnosed by:**
    a. Chest X-ray.
    b. Transillumination.
    c. Percussion and auscultation.
    d. Observation of the chest movement.

12. **A neonate with an Apgar score of 8:**
    a. Requires vigorous resuscitation.
    b. Requires suctioning, oxygen, and positive pressure ventilation only.
    c. Requires cardiac massage, and positive pressure ventilation only.
    d. Requires little, if any, resuscitation.

13. **If a drainage collection system becomes disconnected from a chest tube, what action should be taken immediately?**
    a. Instill sterile saline into the chest tube.
    b. Clamp the chest tube.
    c. Remove the suction from the drainage container.
    d. Attach the suction directly to the chest tube.

Answers for Chapter 17. . . . .

1. Cardiopulmonary status of infants at birth
2. Gestational age of an infant at birth
3. b
4. a
5. b
6. a
7. a

8. a
9. d
10. a
11. a
12. d
13. b

Chapter 18 Questions . . . .

1. Risk factors pointing toward the likelihood of respiratory distress syndrome (RDS) of the neonate include:

    I. Prematurity
    II. Low birth weight
    III. Maternal diabetes
    IV. Second born twin

    a. I, II, and III only
    b. II, III, and IV only
    c. I and II only
    d. I, II, III, and IV

2. Drugs used to produce tocolysis include:

    I. Terbutaline
    II. Magnesium sulfate
    III. Epinephrine
    IV. Vercuronium

    a. I, II, and III only
    b. II, III, and IV only
    c. I and II only
    d. I, II, III, and IV

3. A neonate with a heart rate of 86, peripheral cyanosis, a weak cry, slight flexion of extremities and minimal response to stimulation would have an Apgar score of:

    a. 1
    b. 3
    c. 5
    d. 7

4. Which of the following would NOT be indicated for the treatment of RDS of the newborn?

    a. Endotracheal intubation
    b. Time-cycled pressure-limited ventilation
    c. Continuous positive airway pressure (CPAP)
    d. Cool mist humidification

5. Complicating pathologies commonly seen with RDS of the newborn include:

    I. Pulmonary interstitial emphysema
    II. Patent ductus arteriosis
    III. Pneumothorax or pneumomediastinum
    IV. Meconium aspiration

    a. I, II, III, and IV
    b. I, II, and III only
    c. II, III, and IV only
    d. I and III only

6. Pulmonary surfactant is produced by _____ cells in the lungs.

7. Surfactant begins to appear in the lungs at about _____ weeks' gestation.

8. The administration of _____ to the mother about 48 hours before birth may stimulate surfactant development in the fetus.

9. The nasal flaring seen in infants with RDS of the newborn is probably an attempt to reduce _____.

10. The grunting during exhalation that is seen in infants with RDS of the newborn is probably an attempt to _____

    _____.

11. The possibility of surfactant insufficiency is indicated by a lecithin:sphyngomylin ratio of _____ in amniotic fluid.

12. The apnea of prematurity and thermoregulation problems seen in premature neonates are both probably due to _____

    _____.

13. Premature lungs have (increased/decreased) surface area available for gas exchange compared to mature lungs.

14. The typical "see-saw" breathing pattern seen in premature infants with RDS is due to (compliant/noncompliant) lungs and a (compliant/noncompliant) chest wall.

15. Infants may attempt to maintain body heat by metabolizing (brown fat/white fat) body stores which (increases/decreases) oxygen consumption.

16. Administration of exogenous surfactant is an attempt to (increase/decrease) the compliance of the lungs.

Answers for Chapter 18 . . . .

1. d
2. c
3. c
4. d
5. b
6. Type II pneumocyte
7. 26 weeks
8. Corticosteroids
9. Airway resistance
10. Maintain inflation of alveoli; maintain continuous airway pressure (CPAP)
11. Less than 2:1
12. Immature development of the central nervous system
13. Decreased
14. Noncompliant lung; compliant chest wall
15. Brown fat; increases
16. Increases

Chapter 19 *Questions* . . . .

1. Respiratory damage in a burn victim may be caused by inhaling:
    - I.   Heated gases
    - II. Toxic vapors
    - III. Particulate matter

    a. I and II only
    b. II and III only
    c . I and III only
    d. I, II, and III

2. In a house fire, which of the following toxic substances are likely to be found?
    a. Carbon monoxide
    b. Hydrogen cyanide gas
    c. Formaldehyde
    d. All of the above

3. In the early phases of treating a burn victim, which of the following are major concerns?
    - I.   Abnormalities of oxygen transport
    - II. Thermal injury of the lower airways
    - III. Chemical injury of the lower airways
    - IV. Hypovolemic shock

    a. I, II, and III only
    b. II, III, and IV only
    c. I, III, and IV only
    d. I, II, III, and IV

4. Circumferential burns of the neck and trunk are a concern to RCPs because:
    - I.   Resulting edema may impinge on laryngeal and tracheal patency.
    - II. Thoracic tissues become less elastic and interfere with chest movement.
    - III. Diaphragmatic nerves may be damaged.

    a. I and II only
    b. II and III only
    c. I and III only
    d. I, II, and III

5. Which of the following is true concerning fluid balance in early treatment of burn victims?
    - I.   Loss of fluid creates cardiovascular instability.
    - II. Fluid resuscitation may result in congestive heart failure.
    - III. Intravascular coagulation may compromise circulation.

    a. I and II only
    b. II and III only
    c. I and III only
    d. I, II, and III

6. **The use of pulse oximetry in burn victims:**
    a. Provides the most rapid assessment of oxygenation status available.
    b. Is not dependable because of the presence of carbaminohemoglobin.
    c. Usually correlates well with co-oximetry.
    d. Is not dependable because of the presence of carboxyhemoglobin.

7. **The most reliable index of oxygenation status in burn victims is:**
    a. Arterial oxygen content (CaO_2)
    b. Arterial oxygen tension (PaO_2)
    c. Pulse oximetry (SpO_2)
    d. Venous oxygen tension (PvO_2)

8. **The inhalation of hydrogen cyanide gas during a fire creates problems with:**
    a. The ability of hemoglobin to transport oxygen.
    b. The ability of tissues to use oxygen.
    c. The ability of oxygen to diffuse across the alveolar capillary membrane.
    d. All of the above.

9. **The early respiratory treatment of burn victims should include:**
    a. Administration of an F_IO_2 of 100%.
    b. Hyperbaric oxygenation during transport to the hospital.
    c. Maintaining a PaO_2 of 90ñ100 mm Hg.
    d. Avoiding oxygen induced hypoventilation.

10. **Respiratory problems that do not develop until 36–72 hours after burn injury include:**
    I.   Increased carbon dioxide production due to the development of a hypermetabolic state.
    II. Small airway obstruction from mucosal debris.
    III. Secretion retention from damage to the mucocillary system.
    IV. Decreased oxygen transport capability due to a decrease in circulating red blood cells.

    a. I, II, and III only
    b. I, II, and IV only
    c. II, III, and IV only
    d. I, II, III, and IV

11. **Respiratory infections become a major problem in burn victims because:**
    a. Mucocilliary clearance mechanisms are not functioning properly.
    b. There is immune suppression from the burns.
    c. The patient is not able to cough effectively.
    d. All of the above.

12. **Measurement of hemodynamic parameters via Swan-Ganz catheter is valuable in the management of burn victims because:**
    a. It provides continuous monitoring of systemic blood pressure.
    b. It aids in determining oxygen needs.
    c. It aids in maintaining appropriate fluid balance.
    d. All of the above.

13. **Hyperbaric oxygen therapy benefits burn victims by:**
    I.   Increasing oxygen transport.
    II. Increasing the rate of carbon monoxide excretion.

III. Helping to prevent anaerobic infections.

a. I and II only
b. II and III only
c. I and III only
d. I, II, and III

14. **The nutritional requirements of burn victims are best determined by:**

a. The use of nomograms
b. Daily weighing of the patient
c. Daily electrolyte and blood protein measurements
d. Indirect calorimetry

15. **List at least five goals of respiratory care for patients who are burn victims.**

_____

_____

_____

_____

_____

_____

Answers for Chapter 19 . . . .

1. d

2. d

3. c

4. a

5. d

6. d

7. a

8. b

9. a

10. d

11. d

12. c

13. d

14. d

15. Maintain a patent airway

Maintain effective ventilation

Maintain adequate oxygenation

Maintain adequate acid-base balance

Maintain lung volumes

Suppress infections

Maintain cardiovascular stability